IFMBE Proceedings 90

Series Editor

The IFMBE Proceedings Book Series is an official publication of *the International Federation for Medical and Biological Engineering* (IFMBE). The series gathers the proceedings of various international conferences, which are either organized or endorsed by the Federation. Books published in this series report on cutting-edge findings and provide an informative survey on the most challenging topics and advances in the fields of medicine, biology, clinical engineering, and biophysics.

The series aims at disseminating high quality scientific information, encouraging both basic and applied research, and promoting world-wide collaboration between researchers and practitioners in the field of Medical and Biological Engineering.

Topics include, but are not limited to:

- Diagnostic Imaging, Image Processing, Biomedical Signal Processing
- Modeling and Simulation, Biomechanics
- Biomaterials, Cellular and Tissue Engineering
- Information and Communication in Medicine, Telemedicine and e-Health
- Instrumentation and Clinical Engineering
- Surgery, Minimal Invasive Interventions, Endoscopy and Image Guided Therapy
- Audiology, Ophthalmology, Emergency and Dental Medicine Applications
- Radiology, Radiation Oncology and Biological Effects of Radiation

IFMBE proceedings are indexed by SCOPUS, EI Compendex, Japanese Science and Technology Agency (JST), SCImago. They are also submitted for consideration by WoS.

Proposals can be submitted by contacting the Springer responsible editor shown on the series webpage (see "Contacts"), or by getting in touch with the series editor Ratko Magjarevic.

Petra Bonačić Bartolin · Ratko Magjarević ·
Matthew Allen · Michael Sutcliffe
Editors

Advances in Biomedical and Veterinary Engineering

Selected Contributions to the 1st European Congress on Biomedical and Veterinary Engineering, BioMedVetMech 2022, October 1–3, 2022, Zagreb, Croatia

Springer

Editors
Petra Bonačić Bartolin
Department of Mechanical Engineering,
The Biomechanics Group
Imperial College London
London, UK

Ratko Magjarević
Faculty of Electrical Engineering
and Computing
University of Zagreb
Zagreb, Croatia

Matthew Allen
Department of Veterinary Medicine
University of Cambridge
Cambridge, UK

Michael Sutcliffe
Engineering Department
University of Cambridge
Cambridge, UK

ISSN 1680-0737 ISSN 1433-9277 (electronic)
IFMBE Proceedings
ISBN 978-3-031-42242-3 ISBN 978-3-031-42243-0 (eBook)
https://doi.org/10.1007/978-3-031-42243-0

This Springer imprint is published by the registered company Springer Nature Switzerland AG
The registered company address is: Gewerbestrasse 11, 6330 Cham, Switzerland

Preface

Dear readers, scientists, engineers and doctors, colleagues, and collaborators

In the past fifty years, the use of engineering in human and veterinary medicine has transformed and enhanced the field of patient care. Biomedical and veterinary engineering covers several specialisations and scientific fields such as biomechanics, biomaterials, but also other subdisciplines including the design and development of medical devices, orthopaedic implants, medical imaging, biomedical signal processing, tissue and stem cell engineering, rehabilitation, and clinical engineering. In a multidisciplinary team, experts from the fields—including scientists, mechanical engineers, physicists, doctors, and practitioners—solve challenging medical and veterinary problems. To keep conducting research and create innovations in this area that benefit both people and animals and improve their quality of life, it is essential to offer gratitude to everyone who has contributed. One key tool for bringing these same experts together in one place to realise new collaborations and new projects and publish academic papers whose outcomes are crucial for the advancement of this field is the **1st European Congress on Biomedical and Veterinary Engineering-BioMedVetMech**. This proceedings presents some of the key and ongoing research topics across a few biomedical and veterinary engineering fields. These works illustrated how the collaboration of many professions allowed for the development of novel and distinctive approaches to treating medical and veterinary problems.

Finally, we thank all the authors who contributed to this 1st European Congress on Biomedical and Veterinary Engineering Proceedings issue.

July 2023

Petra Bonačić Bartolin
BioMedVetMech 2022,
Conference Chair

Organisation

Conference Chair

Petra Bonačić Bartolin, Zagreb, Croatia

Conference Co-chairs

Matthew J. Allen, Cambridge, UK
Hrvoje Gasparović, Zagreb, Croatia
Michael Sutcliffe, Cambridge, UK
Ratko Magjarević, Zagreb, Croatia
Vida Demarin, Zagreb, Croatia

Local Organising Committee

Petra Bonačić Bartolin, Zagreb, Croatia
Matthew J. Allen, Cambridge, UK
Michael Sutcliffe, Cambridge, UK
Ratko Magjarević, Zagreb, Croatia
Vida Demarin, Zagreb, Croatia
Brankica Gudeljević, Zagreb, Croatia

Conference Webpage

http://www.biomedvetmech.com/

Croatian Society for Orthopaedic Engineering, Zagreb, Croatia

The Croatian Society for Orthopaedic Engineering is a non-profit organisation established in 2018 in Zagreb, Croatia, that brings together professionals in human and veterinary medicine, engineering, and research. The association's main goals are to promote, develop, and improve orthopaedic services and products, as well as to promote innovation in the field of orthopaedic engineering.

The association also recognised the value of fostering education and training members to gain technical, technological, and information technology knowledge and skills in the field of orthopaedics and orthopaedic engineering www.orthoing.com.

Biomedvetmech 2023 Was Endorsed by:

International Federation for Medical and Biological Engineering (IFMBE)
Surgical Discovery Centre, University of Cambridge, Cambridge
Ministry of Science and Education, Zagreb, Croatia
University of Zagreb, Zagreb, Croatia
Ministry of Health, Zagreb, Croatia
Croatian Biomedical Engineering and Medical Physics Society

Sponsors

Arthrex Adria d.o.o., Zagreb, Croatia
Emma servis, d.o.o., Zagreb, Croatia
Zagreb Tourist Board, Zagreb, Croatia
VamsTec, Zagreb, Croatia

Contents

Influence of *In Vitro* Cultivation on Differentiation Gene Expressions in Canine Adipose-Derived Mesenchymal Stem Cells 1
Marina Prišlin, Dunja Vlahović, Ivana Ljolje, Petar Kostešić, Nenad Turk, Šimun Naletilić, Dragan Brnić, and Nina Krešić

Brain Computer Interface in Neurology: The Future of Neurorestoration, the Possibilities and Perils. A Narrative Review 19
Slaven Lasić, Filip Đerke, Silvio Bašić, and Vida Demarin

High Wall Shear Stress and Its Gradient Indicates Intimal Hyperplasia in Vascular Bypass Graft End-to-Side Distal Anastomosis 35
Severino Krizmanić, Dino Papeš, Predrag Pavić, and Zdravko Virag

Non-invasive Functional Electrical Stimulation in Rehabilitation Engineering ... 46
Lana Popović-Maneski

Low-Back Pain Patients Classification Based on sEMG Activation Patterns Detection 53
Vedran Srhoj-Egekher, Mario Cifrek, and Stanislav Peharec

Wireless Device for Biomedical Signal Acquisition with Dry Electrodes on an e-Bike 60
L. Klaić, I. Čuljak, A. Stanešić, I. Vrhoci, P. Šajinović, M. Cifrek, and H. Džapo

Automatic Objective Magnification Detection in Brightfield Microscopy by Use of Neural Network 73
Dora Machaček and Ivan-Conrado Šoštarić-Zuckermann

Virtual Surgery and 3D Printing in Craniofacial Surgery – Our Experience at UHC Osijek Using a Newly Developed Add-On for "Open-Source" 3D Modeling Software 81
Vjekoslav Kopačin, Ivan Mumlek, Vedran Zubčić, Josip Butković, and Luka Šimić

Author Index 89

Influence of *In Vitro* Cultivation on Differentiation Gene Expressions in Canine Adipose-Derived Mesenchymal Stem Cells

Marina Prišlin[1(✉)], Dunja Vlahović[2], Ivana Ljolje[3], Petar Kostešić[4], Nenad Turk[5], Šimun Naletilić[6], Dragan Brnić[1], and Nina Krešić[1]

[1] Virology Department, Croatian Veterinary Institute, Zagreb, Croatia
prislin@veinst.hr

[2] Department of Veterinary Pathology, Faculty of Veterinary Medicine, University of Zagreb, Zagreb, Croatia

[3] Veterinary Clinic for Small Animals Buba, Zagreb, Croatia

[4] Surgery, Orthopaedic and Ophthalmology Clinic, Faculty of Veterinary Medicine, University of Zagreb, Zagreb, Croatia

[5] Department of Microbiology and Infectious Diseases With Clinic, Faculty of Veterinary Medicine, University of Zagreb, Zagreb, Croatia

[6] Department for Pathological Morphology, Croatian Veterinary Institute, Zagreb, Croatia

Abstract. Canine adipose-derived mesenchymal stem cells (cAD-MSCs) have been demonstrated to be effective in treating several illnesses due to, among others, their differentiation (DI) potential. However, some treatments require *in vitro* multiplication of cAD-MSCs, which may alter their DI characteristics. This research aimed to determine if *in vitro* cultivation affects DI processes in the molecular profiles of cAD-MSCs. Isolation of cAD-MSCs from the abdominal adipose tissue of eight young female dogs was performed, and their immunophenotype and *in vitro* DI potential was confirmed. Total RNA was extracted in the early passage (P) 3 and late P6, and changes in the gene expression profile linked to DI were examined using a microarray. Isolated cAD-MSCs arrested proliferation at P8, on average. They displayed typical immunophenotypes and maintained their DI potential during *in vitro* cultivation. Gene up- and downregulations were observed; however, the overall expression was not significantly altered comparing P3 to P6. The obtained results of up- and downregulations suggest *in vitro* cultivation may favour DI events, as indicated by the overexpression of the Growth DI factor 7 (GDF7), a crucial gene for cartilage formation, Kinase insert domain receptor (KDR), a protein involved in angiogenesis during DI, and Fibroblast growth factor 10 (FGF10), a protein required for the development of embryonic limbs. However, T-box transcription factor (TBX5), a promoter of osteoDI and mineralization, was downregulated in P6, suggesting prolonged *in vitro* cultivation could influence the osteoDI potential. The downregulation of Ras Homolog Family Member (RHOA) could be advantageous since overexpression of this gene is linked to the proliferation and spread of malignant cells. More donors and a comparison of the genders should be included in future research. Thus, this research demonstrated that, despite minor alterations, *in vitro* multiplication did not significantly alter the DI potential and gene expression of young female cAD-MSCs, which is a vital prerequisite for producing high-quality canine stem cell products.

P. Bonačić Bartolin et al. (Eds.): BioMedVetMech 2022, IFMBE Proceedings 90, pp. 1–18, 2024.
https://doi.org/10.1007/978-3-031-42243-0_1

Keywords: canine adipose-derived mesenchymal stem cells · differentiation · gene expression · *in vitro* cultivation · microarray

1 Introduction

Mesenchymal stem cells (MSCs) are stromal cells originating from the mesoderm and can regenerate our bodies by replacing cells that have naturally died. These regenerative cells can be found in skeletal muscle [1], umbilical cord blood [2], dental pulp [3], placenta [4], amniotic membrane [5] and others, but the main sources in regenerative medicine are bone marrow [6] and adipose tissue [7]. Adipose-derived MSCs (AD-MSCs) are the most easily isolated with minimal risk to the donor, so their features in regenerative medicine are highly investigated. The first successful isolation of AD-MSCs from canines was made in 2008, but the exact mechanism by which these cells regenerate tissues is yet unknown. It is known that they can detect injured tissues, produce beneficial immunomodulatory chemicals, and develop into different cell types [8, 9]. Canine AD-MSCs (cAD-MSCs) can differentiate into adipocytes, osteocytes, myocytes, and chondrocytes [10], and recently the ability of differentiation (DI) in a neuronal lineage has been explored [11, 12].

In terms of therapy, cAD-MSCs have been demonstrated to be successful in treating orthopaedic [13], dermatology [14], ophthalmology [15], neurology [16], gastrointestinal [17], and hepatology [18] pathologies. However, a large number of cAD-MSCs are necessary for the successful treatment of some diseases. Thus, before being used in clinical settings, *in vitro* expansion is required due to the restricted amount of cAD-MSCs in tissue. Such laboratory manipulation may impact the characteristics of cAD-MSCs and their capacity to differentiate into various cell types [19]. The results obtained by differentiating four subpassages revealed that cAD-MSCs exhibit a decrease in osteogenic differentiation (DI) during *in vitro* cultivation [20]. Furthermore, expression of DI genes, such as lipoprotein lipase (LPL), was significantly lower in older dogs, which means that even though the DI potential of cells is retained, it is decreasing with age [21, 22]. In the study of bovine AD-MSCs, long-term *in vitro* expansion had a negative effect on adipogenic and chondrogenic DI, while potentially favoring osteogenesis [23]. On the other hand, research on human AD-MSCs concluded that adipogenic potential might be better preserved over osteogenesis in aged AD-MSCs, suggesting that early passages must be used to preserve osteogenic DI [24].

The capacity of the cell to keep its DI potential throughout *in vitro* cultivation is essential for the regeneration of injured cells, tissues, and organs since multipotency is one of the proposed modes of action in stem cell therapy. Therefore, the unknown DI process changes during *in vitro* cultivation directed the aim of this study in exploring the existence of DI alterations of cAD-MSCs on a molecular level.

2 Material and Methods

2.1 Ethics

The animal protocols used in this work were evaluated and approved by the Veterinary Ethics Committee of the Faculty of Veterinary Medicine of the University of Zagreb, approval code 640–01/20–17/10, February 20th 2020, and 640–01/20–17/55, September 28th 2020 and Ethics Board of the Croatian Veterinary Institute, approval code Z-IV-4–2022/19, May 9th 2019. All canine donors participating in this study were given written informed agreements by their owners before their pets' biological samples were used for research.

2.2 Animals

The study included eight healthy female canine donors (*Canis lupus familiaris)* up to 38 months of age who underwent elective surgical procedures. Table 1 outlines the donors' age, breed, state of health, and surgical technique.

Table 1. Donor information.

Donor	Age (Months)	Breed	Surgical procedure	Origin of adipose tissue	Health status before the procedure
5/20	14,5	Ridgeback	Bilateral ovariectomy	Periovarian area	No detectable signs of illness
7/20	9	Mixed breed	Bilateral ovariectomy	Periovarian area	No detectable signs of illness
8/20	9	Beagle	Bilateral ovariectomy	Ligament falciform	No detectable signs of illness
13/20	38	Mixed breed	Bilateral ovariectomy	Ligament falciform	No detectable signs of illness
6/21	12	German pointer	Ovariohysterectomy	Periovarian area	No detectable signs of illness
9/21	12	Labrador retriever	Bilateral ovariectomy	Periovarian area	No detectable signs of illness
13/21	7	Toy poodle	Bilateral ovariectomy	Periovarian area	No detectable signs of illness
14/21	7	Toy poodle	Bilateral ovariectomy	Periovarian area	No detectable signs of illness

2.3 Adipose Tissue Collection

The collection of adipose tissue was carried out per our prior established protocol [25]. Briefly, the dogs were sedated and an ovariectomy or ovariohysterectomy was performed.

Subsequently, 1–10 g of adipose tissue was collected from biomedical waste in a sterile Falcon tube (without medium) and placed at 4 °C until transport to the laboratory.

2.4 cAD-MSCs Isolation and Cultivation

Within two hours of sampling, an isolation process was applied to all acquired samples. Utilizing 1–10 g of abdominal adipose tissue for mechanical and enzymatic digestion, gained stromal vascular fraction was placed in T25 cell culture flasks (Nunc, ThermoFisher Scientific, Waltham, MA, USA) with basal media. The isolation and cultivation of cAD-MSCs were carried out in accordance with the protocol we previously published [25, 26].

2.5 Differentiation Assay

As previously reported [25], following the The International Society for Cellular Therapy (ISCT) guidelines [27], trilineage DI (adipogenic, osteogenic, and chondrogenic) was conducted in the third passage (P3) confirming that isolated cAD-MSCs can differentiate. In brief, cells were seeded in a basal medium of the 24-microwell plate (Nunc, ThermoFisher Scientific, Waltham, MA, USA) in triplicate. When cells had reached confluence after 48 h, the medium was changed to 1 mL of StemMACS AdipoDiff media for adipoDI or StemMACS OsteoDiff media for osteoDI (both from Miltenyi Biotec, Bergisch Gladbach, Germany). In addition, control wells were grown in basal media. Every 48 to 72 h, DI and basal media were changed. Using ChondroDiff Media (Miltenyi Biotec, Bergisch Gladbach, Germany), ChondroDI was conducted for 21 days in 15 mL conical polypropylene tubes in spheroid form, while the control tube was left in basal media. Plates and tubes were incubated at 37 °C, 5% CO2, and 95% humidity with the tube lids slightly opened. Every 48 to 72 h, the media were replaced.

The procedures described in a recent publication [25] were used to detect differentiated adipocytes, osteoblasts, and chondrocytes. AdipoDI staining was carried out using Oil Red O to identify lipid droplets and osteoDI using SIGMAFAST BCIP/NBT substrate to identify alkaline phosphatase activity (both from Sigma-Aldrich, St. Louis, MO, USA). For adipoDI, red-stained cells were deemed affirmative, and for osteoDI, purple-stained cells. After dehydration and paraffin embedding, the presence of chondrocytes in the spheroids was determined. After rehydrating, a 2,5 g staining with Alcian blue 8GX (Sigma-Aldrich, St. Louis, MO, USA) was done to test for aggrecan. Following staining, slides or cells were examined with an Axio Observer D1 inverted microscope and photographs were made using a camera (Total magnification: 50x-200x, Zeiss, Oberkochen, Germany).

2.6 Flow Cytometry Immunophenotyping

To corroborate the stem cell immunophenotype following the International Stem Cell Therapy guidelines [27], the undifferentiated cAD-MSCs were characterized in a P3 using flow cytometry. The requirements were as stated before [25] for the flow cytometry studies performed on the BD FACSVerse (BD Biosciences, Franklin Lakes, NJ, USA).

The developed antibody panel is shown in Table 2. CS&T beads (BD Biosciences, Franklin Lakes, NJ, USA) lot numbers 92323 and 13697 were used for daily performance quality control (QC) before starting each experiment, and characterization QC was carried out every six months.

Table 2. Flow cytometry antibody panel used in this study.

Antigen	Clone	Host	Fluorophore	Reactivity	Clonality	Manufacturer/Catalog number
CD44	MEM-263	Mouse	FITC	Canine, Human, Porcine	Monoclonal	Antibodies-online, Aachen, Germany /ABIN452099
Isotype IgG1	VI-AP	Mouse	FITC		Monoclonal	Antibodies-online, Aachen, Germany /ABIN1741583
CD45	YKIX716.13	Rat	PE	Canine	Monoclonal	Bio-Rad, Hercules, CA, USA /MCA1042PE
Isotype IgG2b		Rat	PE		Monoclonal	Bio-Rad, Hercules, CA, USA /MCA6006PE
CD73		Rabbit	PE	Human, Mouse, Rat, Canine, Chicken	Polyclonal	Bioss antibodies, Woburn, MA, USA /bs-4834R-PE
Isotype IgG		Rabbit	PE		Polyclonal	Antibodies-online, Aachen, Germany /ABIN376422
CD 29	MEM-101A	Mouse	FITC	Canine, Human, Porcine	Monoclonal	Antibodies-online, Aachen, Germany /ABIN94056
Isotype IgG1	VI-AP	Mouse	FITC		Monoclonal	Antibodies-online, Aachen, Germany /ABIN1741583
CD271 (4 donors)	ME20.4–1.H4	Mouse	FITC	Human, Canine	Monoclonal	Miltenyi Biotec, Bergisch Gladbach, Germany /130–098-103
Isotype IgG1	IS5-21F5	Mouse	FITC		Monoclonal	Miltenyi Biotec, Bergisch Gladbach, Germany /130–113-761

(*continued*)

Table 2. (*continued*)

Antigen	Clone	Host	Fluorophore	Reactivity	Clonality	Manufacturer/Catalog number
CD271 (4 donors)	ME20.4	Mouse	APC	Canine, Human, Mouse, Non-human primate, Sheep, Pig, Rabbit, Rat	Monoclonal	Thermo Fisher Scientific, Waltham, MA, USA / 17–9400-42
Isotype IgG1, kappa	P3.6.2.8.1	Mouse	APC		Monoclonal	Thermo Fisher Scientific, Waltham, MA, USA /17–4714-42
CD90	YKIX337.217	Rat	APC	Canine	Monoclonal	Thermo Fisher Scientific, Waltham, MA, USA / 17–5900-42
Isotype IgG2b, kappa	eB149/10H5	Rat	APC		Monoclonal	Thermo Fisher Scientific, Waltham, MA, USA / 17–4031-82
CD14	MφP9	Mouse	PE-Cy 7	Human, Canine	Monoclonal	BD Biosciences, Franklin Lakes, NJ, USA/557742
Isotype IgG2a, kappa	G155–178	Mouse	PE-Cy 7		Monoclonal	BD Biosciences, Franklin Lakes, NJ, USA/557907
CD105	SN6	Mouse	PE-Cy 7	Human, published species canine	Monoclonal	Thermo Fisher Scientific, Waltham, MA, USA /25–1057-42

Antibody Staining

For the cAD-MSCs immunophenotype test, the previously described published technique was followed, and the single stain labelling approach was applied for 10^5 cells per test tube [25]. Unstained cells were used to calibrate the experimental conditions, and identical conditions were applied to each tube throughout each experiment. At the end of the experiment, cell viability was evaluated using a Propidium Iodide staining solution (BD Biosciences, Franklin Lakes, NJ, USA).

Analysis

All data files have been gated using the same method as previously reported [25]. A homogenous population was chosen using the first gate, duplicate cells were excluded using the second gate, and dead cells were excluded using the third gate on the propidium iodide test tube. FACSuite software (BD Biosciences, Franklin Lakes, NJ, USA) was used to analyze 10,000 collected events, and the results were represented as the median fluorescence intensity (MFI). Apart from CD105, where the MFI antibody was divided with the MFI of unstained cells due to insufficient isotype control for canine cells, MFI fold change was calculated by dividing the median of the relevant antibody with the median of isotype control. The fold change cut-off was set at 1.5.

2.7 Gene Expression Microarray Analysis

Total RNA Extraction

After cAD-MSC reached 80–90% confluence in T75 cell culture flasks (Nunc, ThermoFisher Scientific, Waltham, MA, USA) at P3 and P6, total RNA was extracted from the cells. A cell scraper was used to detach the cells, which were then centrifuged at 235 g for 10 min. Next, total RNA was extracted using the RNeasy Mini Kit (Qiagen, Hilden, Germany), as directed by the manufacturer. Also, according to the manufacturer's instructions, the QIAxcel RNA QC Kit (Qiagen, Germany) was used on the QIAxcel Advanced device for capillary electrophoresis for assessing the RNA integrity number (RIN) and concentration of isolated RNAs. Utilizing an Implen Nanophotometer P360 (Munich, Germany), the absorbance of the RNA was measured to evaluate its purity.

Real-Time PCR Array

Following the manufacturer's instructions, changes in the expression of cAD-MSCs genes involved in, among other things, DI events were examined using validated RT2 Profiler PCR Array Format R with SYBR Green-optimized primer assays (Qiagen, Hilden, Germany) compatible for use with Rotor-Gene Q. First, using RT2 First Strand Kit (Qiagen, Hilden, Germany) and 800 ng of total RNA as a template, genomic DNA (gDNA) was eliminated and complementary DNA (cDNA) was synthesized according to manufacturer instructions. After that, 20 μL of the mixture containing the SYBR Green primers and the cDNA template was applied to each well. The array has primers designed specifically for the genes ABCB1, BMP2, BMP4, GDF5, GDF7, KAT2B, HAT1, SOX9, ADIPOQ, CEBPD, FASN, INSR, LPL, PPARG, RHOA, RUNX2, FGF10, KDR, HDAC1, PTK2, SMURF1, SMURF2, TBX5 and TGFB1 (Table 3 provides a collection of complete gene names and NCBI sequences). Additionally, three wells contain controls for reverse transcription, three wells contain the PCR controls, and one well is utilized as a gDNA control.

RT2 Profiler PCR Array Data Analysis software, accessible online at https://dataanalysis2.qiagen.com/pcr (accessed on October 3rd, 2022), was used to evaluate the obtained data. Using the Ct method, the software analyzes the data and performs statistical analysis (based on the Student's t-test), which is fully provided in a detailed report; differences in gene expression levels were interpreted as significant if $p < 0.05$. The fold change cut-off was set at 2.

Table 3. Alphabetically listed full names, abbreviations and NCBI reference sequences of investigated genes.

Gene name	Gene abbreviation	NCBI RefSeq
Adiponectin gene	ADIPOQ	NM_001006644
ATP binding cassette subfamily B member 1	ABCB1	NM_001003215
Bone morphogenetic protein 2	BMP2	XM_534351
Bone morphogenetic protein 4	BMP4	NM_001287170
CCAAT enhancer binding protein delta	CEBPD	XM_843188
Fatty acid synthase	FASN	XM_005624145
Fibroblast growth factor 10	FGF10	XM_005619337
Growth differentiation factor 5	GDF5	XM_542974
Growth differentiation factor 7	GDF7	XM_540103
Histone acetyltransferase 1	HAT1	XM_005640309
Histone deacetylase 1	HDAC1	XM_544435
Insulin receptor	INSR	XM_005633222
Lysine acetyltransferase 2B	KAT2B	XM_014106497
Kinase insert domain receptor	KDR	NM_001048024
Lipoprotein lipase	LPL	XM_005635734
Peroxisome proliferator-activated receptor gamma	PPARG	NM_001024632
Protein tyrosine kinase	PTK2	XM_005627993
Ras homolog family member A	RHOA	NM_001003273
Runt-related transcription factor 2	RUNX2	XM_005642335
SMAD specific E3 ubiquitin protein ligase 1	SMURF1	XM_005621177
SMAD specific E3 ubiquitin protein ligase 2	SMURF2	XM_537589
SRY-Box transcription factor 9	SOX9	NM_001002978
T-box transcription factor	TBX5	XM_548568
Transforming growth factor beta 1	TGFB1	NM_001003309

2.8 Statistics

The Whisker box plot was used for presenting the minimum, maximum, median, and quartiles of MFI fold change values of each marker in the flow cytometry results graphically (GraphPad Prism, version 9.4.1.). The RT2 Profiler PCR Array Data Analysis software using the Student's t-test was used to statistically verify the results of the microarray gene expression analysis ($p < 0.05$).

3 Results

3.1 cAD-MSCs Isolation and Cultivation

All donors' cAD-MSC cultures were successfully established as a result of the isolation protocol that was used. Spindle-shaped isolated cells underwent *in vitro* cultivation, increased their size and granularity, and decreased their density due to senescence, i.e. morphological alterations between early (P3) and late (P6) passage were seen using a live cell analysis platform (Fig. 1; Cytosmart Lux2, CytoSMART Technologies B.V., Eindhoven, Netherlands). Proliferation stopped at P8 on average; however, donor 13/21 had a remarkable capacity for proliferating and reached P12.

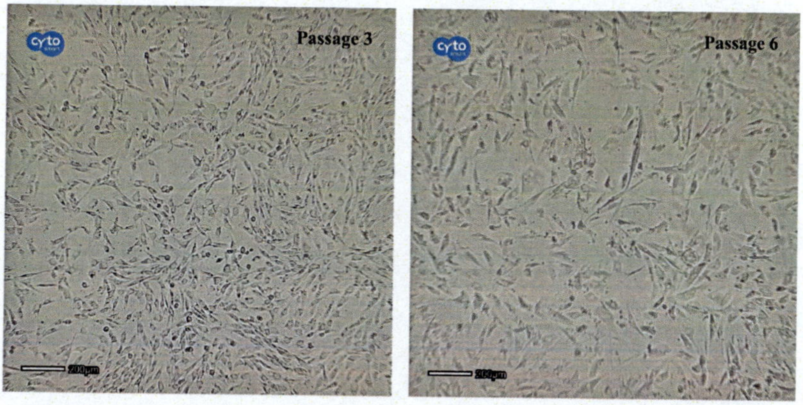

Fig. 1. Morphological differences of canine adipose-derived mesenchymal stem cells representative donor 9/21 cultivated *in vitro*, passage 3 and passage 6. Pictures were obtained with live cell analysis platform Cytosmart Lux2 (CytoSMART Technologies B.V., Eindhoven, Netherlands).

3.2 Differentiation Assay

The trilineage (adipogenic, osteogenic, and chondrogenic) DI capacity *in vitro* was preserved in P3, and the isolated cells have been confirmed to have a differentiation capacity according to ISCT criteria. However, osteoDI intensity was lowered when the monolayered cells began forming a spheroidal shape. Pictures of the adipoDI (Fig. 2A-B), osteoDI (Fig. 2C-D), and chondroDI (Fig. 2D-F) DI results from the 13/20 donor experiment are displayed.

3.3 Flow Cytometry Immunophenotype Characterization

Isolated cAD-MSCs in P3 underwent flow cytometry analysis, which revealed the presence of CD90, CD105, CD44, CD29, and present but low CD73 (MFI fold change average = 1.5), confirming the isolated cells' stem cell status following ISCT guidelines. CD271, CD45, and CD14 expressions were not found. The calculated MFI fold changes for all CD markers are displayed as a dotted whisker-box plot in Fig. 3, where the individual data are represented by the different-colored triangles.

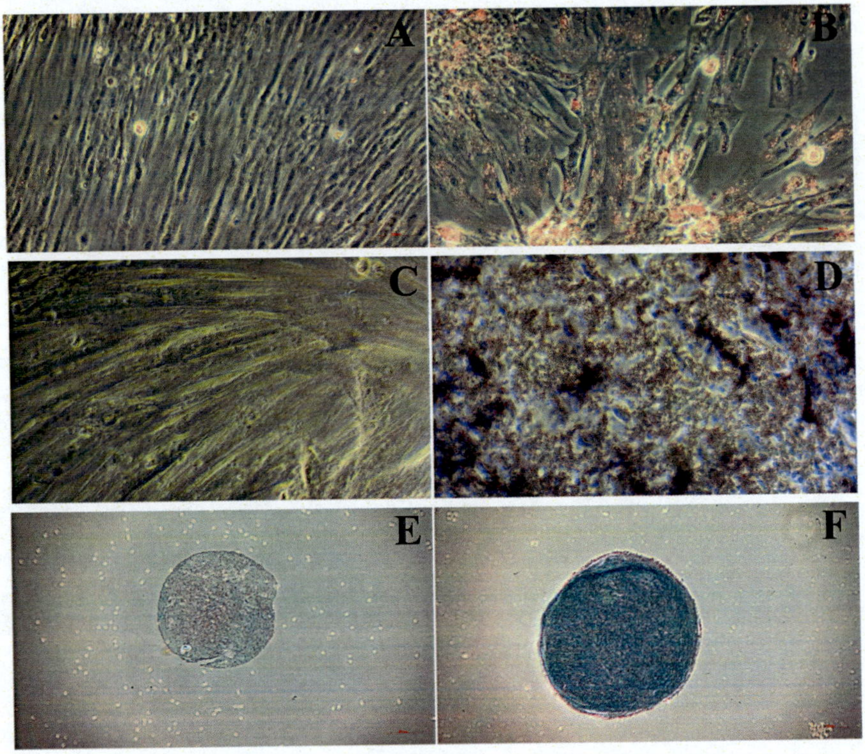

Fig. 2. The functionality of canine adipose-derived mesenchymal stem cells (cAD-MSCs) is demonstrated by successful adipo-, osteo- and chondro- differentiation (DI). (2A-B) Microscopic images (100 ×) of cAD-MSCs after adipoDI stained with Oil O Red for detection of lipid droplets within the cell. Cells cultivated in basal medium (negative control) showed a lack of red staining. (2A), and cAD-MSCs cultivated in StemMACS AdipoDiff Media (Miltenyi Biotec, Bergisch Gladbach, Germany) showed high-intensity red staining of accumulated lipid droplets within the cell (2B). (2C-D) Microscopic images (200 ×) of cAD-MSCs after osteoDI stained with SIGMAFAST™ BCIP (R)/NTB substrate (Sigma-Aldrich, St. Louis, MO, Germany) to detect alkaline phosphatase activity. Cells cultivated in basal medium (negative control) showed low-intensity staining. (2C) cAD-MSCs cultivated in StemMACS OsteoDiff Media (Miltenyi Biotec, Bergisch Gladbach, Germany) showed high-intensity staining for alkaline phosphatase activity (2D). (2E) Microscopic images (50x) of spheroids cultivated in basal medium (negative control) stained with Alcian blue showing a lack of staining for aggrecan of the extracellular matrix (ECM). (2F) Spheroids grown in StemMACS ChondroDiff Media (Miltenyi Biotec, Bergisch Gladbach, Germany), stained with Alcian Blue, showing staining for ECM aggrecan. Microscopic pictures were taken with an Axiovert camera on the Axio Observer D1 microscope (Zeiss, Oberkochen, Germany).

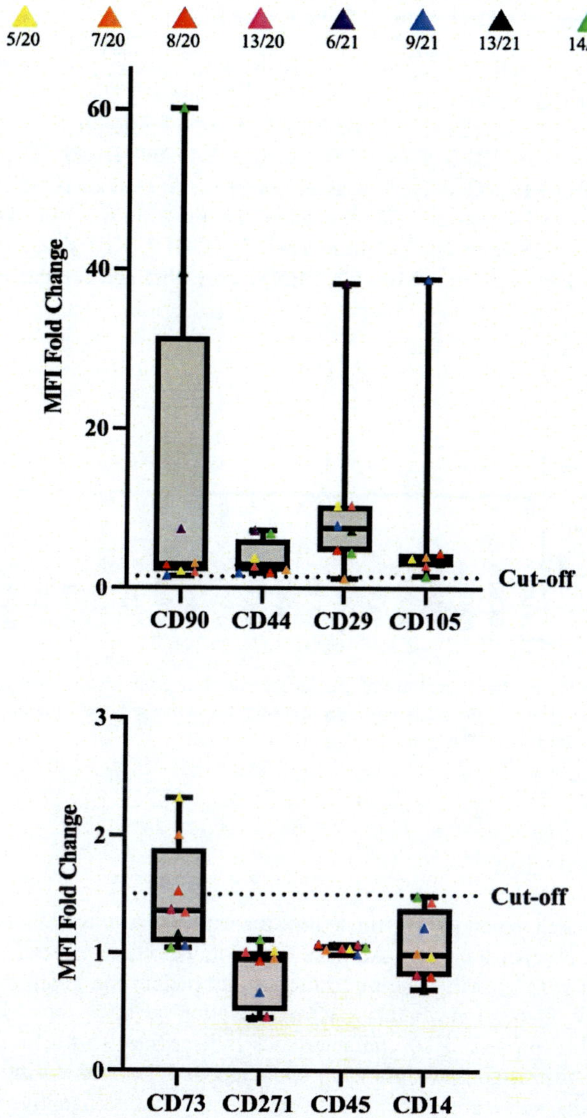

Fig. 3. Whisker-box plot representation of Median fluorescence intensity (MFI) fold changes in canine adipose-derived mesenchymal stem cells for surface markers CD90, CD44, CD29, CD105 (box plot above), CD73, CD271, CD45 and CD14 (box plot below) in the third passage. The cut-off value of 1.5 is represented by the dotted line, and colorful triangles represent the individual MFI fold change values for each donor in the legend above.

3.4 Microarray Detection of Gene Expression

All donors' total RNA was successfully extracted, and an analysis of the RNA integrity number (RIN) revealed that it ranged from 10.0 to 8.9, indicating that the RNA was of high quality. Furthermore, analysis of DI gene expression markers (ADIPOQ, ABCB1, BMP2, BMP4, CEBPD, FASN, FGF10, GDF5, GDF7, HAT1, HDAC1, INSR, KAT2B, KDR, LPL, PPARG, PTK2, RHOA, RUNX2, SOX9, SMURF1, SMURF2, TBX5, TGFB1) revealed that the overall change in expression was not statistically significant. Although three gene upregulations (FGF10, GDF7, KDR) and five downregulations (HDAC1, LPL, RHOA, SMURF2, TBX5) were obtained comparing P6 to P3 (Fig. 4).

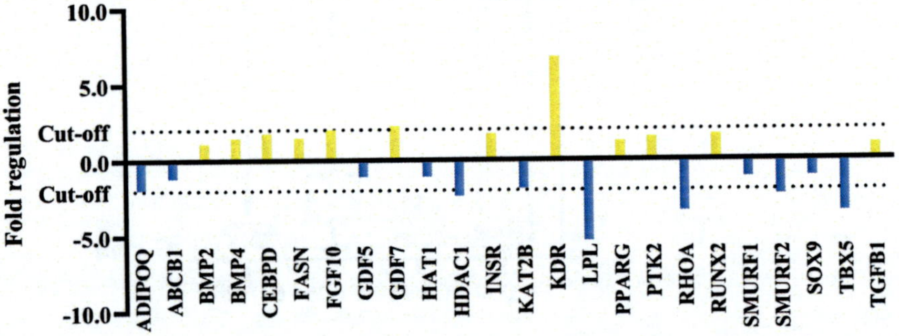

Fig. 4. Fold regulation values of the differentiation gene expression analysis comparing the sixth passage with the third passage cAD-MSCs. Upregulated genes are marked yellow and downregulated blue. The cut-off value is 2.

4 Discussion

This research aimed to investigate how the expression of the DI genes changed as cAD-MSCs were grown *in vitro*. Adipose tissue only contains a small number of stem cells; hence *in vitro* growth is required to give the patient the greatest treatment outcomes. Therefore, finding out whether *in vitro* cultivation can affect the cAD-MSCs regeneration in terms of preserved DI characteristics is necessary to fill the knowledge gap. Our findings suggested that significant spontaneous DI events during cultivation were not present since *in vitro* exploitation did not statistically significantly change the DI potential in young female cAD-MSCs, comparing the third, as early, and sixth, as late passage, respectively. However, there have been up- and downregulations in the expression of DI genes, which should not be ignored straightaway.

Eight young female dogs cAD-MSCs were examined in this study to assess the impact of *in vitro* adaptation on certain genes implicated in the DI process. The explored cells showed plastic adherence and were spindle-shaped, which aligns with ISCT criteria for stem cells [27]. One donor had a high proliferation capacity, indicating donors' proliferation individuality. Since the cAD-MSCs from this donor where extracted from only 1 g of adipose tissue, suggestively, the weight of the tissue is not correlated with the proliferation capacity, but the influence of age, gender, and breed on proliferation capacity should be further explored. Young donor cAD-MSCs had a much higher cumulative population doubling level than older donor cAD-MSCs, which Lee et al. theorized was caused by age-related telomeric shortening [22]. Selle and his colleagues also discovered a gender difference in human bone marrow MSCs, with females having a lower proliferative ability than males[28]. Additionally, the shift in cell morphology that has been demonstrated is a sign of molecular-level changes. Numerous research teams have already established that MSCs cultivated *in vitro* can undergo morphological, phenotypic, and genetic alterations regardless of the culture medium [24, 29]. When comparing early to late Ps, the identified genetic changes entailed a significant decrease in fold change, particularly in the genes associated with DI characteristics, such as LPL, PPARG, and RUNX2 [24]. This result suggested a direction for additional research on the impact of *in vitro* cultivation on the expression of DI genes.

Although the DI media utilized in this study for functionality testing are designed for human use, they can still distinguish cAD-MSCs when employed following our slightly modified technique, as shown in this study and our earlier research [25], which was also confirmed by another research team [30]. While osteogenic DI identified with the alkaline phosphatase detection substrate revealed the low-intensity-stained activity of this enzyme, adipogenic and chondrogenic DI was highly intense. One of the causes might be the spheroids that spontaneously form during osteoDI and are difficult to stain, as observed by other research groups [8, 31, 32]. After labelling cAD-MSCs with Alizarin Red S for calcium deposit detection, Rashid and colleagues showed cell dissociation but successful DI staining of osteocytes [32]. Mineral deposits were effectively stained with Alizarin Red S in another DI investigation of cAD-MSCs, therefore, this kind of staining should be considered in our future studies [33].

Characterization of cAD-MSCs was carried out in a P3 to confirm the stem cell immunophenotype. The created antibody panel for flow cytometry experiments resulted in well-measured expression of selected markers CD90^{+}, CD44^{+}, CD29^{+} and CD105^{+}, except in the case of CD73^{+}, which is the only polyclonal antibody in the panel. Regarding CD73, in a study of murine MSCs, CD73^{high+} MSCs were found beneficial for their reparative properties and anti-inflammatory activity in cardiac repair in comparison to CD73^{low+} [34]. Considering the importance of CD73 expression, a more suitable antibody is needed. Takemitsu et al. [35] observed the same surface protein expression, and similar results have been found by Screven et al. [21], but apart from CD29, where cAD-MSCs continuously showed high percentage positivity [25, 26]. That is an expected finding since CD29 is highly expressed by adipocyte progenitors [36]. CD45 and CD14 were found negative, consistent with our previous research, but a slight difference in CD271 was found, probably due to the certain heterogeneity of the cells in the early Ps [25].

Changes in DI genes between P3 and P6 were investigated, respectively, as immunophenotype and DI functionality testing were conducted to identify adherent cells as stem cells. Since published studies show inconsistent results regarding DI potential in aged *in vitro* cultured AD-MSCs [20, 23, 24], there is a great need for further research. A commercially available validated microarray kit for assessing cAD-MSCs gene expression was employed to ensure consistency throughout this study and simplicity in comparing the findings with others in future. The primers in this kit target 89 MSC-related genes; however, the focus of this study was on the following DI genes: ADIPOQ, ABCB1, BMP2, BMP4, CEBPD, FASN, FGF10, GDF5, GDF7, HAT1, HDAC1, INSR, KAT2B, KDR, LPL, PPARG, PTK2, RHOA, RUNX2, SOX9, SMURF1, SMURF2, TBX5, and TGFB1.

In comparative research of human placental MSCs from various stages of pregnancy, genes related to early chondrogenesis (ABCB1, SOX-9, BMP4, GDF5, and GDF7) were well conserved [37]. Similar findings were found in this work; however, GDF7 was overexpressed in aged cAD-MSCs cultured *in vitro*, which may be advantageous in joint regeneration therapy [38]. GDF7 is a crucial coding protein for the production of cartilage and may be used as a stimulant in the processes of tenogenesis, osteogenesis, and adipogenesis, according to a recent study. Due to its multiple-lineage stimulating actions, GDF-7 might be a viable growth factor for the regeneration of the tendon-bone interface [39]. KDR overexpression was another finding with possible benefits. The most crucial stages in tissue regeneration, angiogenesis, vascular development, vascular permeability, and embryonic hematopoiesis, are regulated by the VEGF receptor protein encoded by this gene [40]. FGF10 was also upregulated in our study; however, given that it is essential for limb development and embryogenesis, its overexpression for promoting osteogenesis and regeneration is desired [41].

A study on bone marrow MSCs revealed that mechanical stimulation and therapeutic inhibition of HDAC1 orchestrate the expression of genes involved in osteogenic DI [42]. On the other hand, we observed the downregulation of HDAC1, which may also be advantageous for osteogenesis. Furthermore, data from other authors suggest that the downregulation of HDAC1 is a key process for osteogenesis [43]. Additionally, SMURF2 downregulation is advantageous since it encodes a protein crucial for the interaction and degradation of numerous critical molecules involved in osteogenesis, such as SMAD1 and RUNX2, and it has the potential to adversely affect the osteoDI procedure [44]. On the other hand, since TBX5 and RUNX2 together represent a potent paradigm for the transcriptional regulation of osteogenesis and perhaps other MSCs DI, downregulating TBX5 might be unfavorable [45]. Individually, these data point to a potential impact of prolonged *in vitro* cultivation on the reduced osteoDI potential in our study. Downregulation of LPL was seen in the previous study by Krešić et al. [26]. This research confirms the trend of decreased LPL expression, which can lead to lower adipoDI potential during prolonged *in vitro* culture [46]. The LPL gene encodes a protein needed for the metabolism of fatty acids. Since the cells are ageing, it was anticipated that the RHOA would be downregulated because it encodes Rho GTPases necessary for the remodelling of the actin cytoskeleton and the control of cell shape, adhesion, and motility. The overexpression of the RHOA protein is linked to the proliferation and spread of tumor cells, therefore, this downregulation is equally crucial [47].

In conclusion, cAD-MSCs' multipotency is still a topic of intense investigation since it plays a part in repairing injured cells, tissues, or organs. And in this study, we added to the repository of information regarding cAD-MSCs' capacity for maintaining their multipotency during *in vitro* expansion. Young female cAD-MSCs from P3 and P6 did not significantly vary, according to studies on genes related to the DI process. Although protein composition still needs to be correlated, and molecular alterations were not statistically significant, gene regulations should not be overlooked because they may help estimate final protein expression.

Acknowledgments. We thank Mihaela Stuparić Komušar for her generous help during spheroid preparation and staining.

Funding. This research was funded by Croatian Science Foundation (HRZZ) and performed within Installation Research Project (UIP-2019-04-2178) "Revealing transcriptome and secretome of mesenchymal stem cells" SECRET. We thank HRZZ for supporting our research.

References

1. Qu-Petersen, Z., et al.: Identification of a novel population of muscle stem cells in mice: potential for muscle regeneration. J. Cell Biol. **157**, 851–864 (2002). https://doi.org/10.1083/jcb.200108150
2. Erices, A., Conget, P., Minguell, J.J.: Mesenchymal progenitor cells in the human umbilical cord. Br. J. Haematol. **109**, 235–242 (2000). https://doi.org/10.1007/s00277-004-0918-z
3. Gronthos, S., Mankani, M., Brahim, J., Robey, P.G., Shi, S.: Postnatal human dental pulp stem cells (DPSCs) in vitro and in vivo. Proc. Natl. Acad. Sci. U. S. A. **97**, 13625–13630 (2000). https://doi.org/10.1073/pnas.240309797
4. Miao, Z., et al.: Isolation of mesenchymal stem cells from human placenta: comparison with human bone marrow mesenchymal stem cells. Cell Biol. Int. **30**, 681–687 (2006). https://doi.org/10.1016/j.cellbi.2006.03.009
5. Alviano, F., et al.: Term amniotic membrane is a high throughput source for multipotent mesenchymal stem cells with the ability to differentiate into endothelial cells in vitro. BMC Dev. Biol. **7**, 1–14 (2007). https://doi.org/10.1186/1471-213X-7-11
6. Friedenstein, A.J., Petrakova, K.V., Kurolesova, A.I., Frolova, G.P.: Heterotopic of bone marrow. Analysis of precursor cells for osteogenic and hematopoietic tissues. Transplantation **6**, 230–247 (1968)
7. Zuk, P.A., et al.: Multilineage cells from human adipose tissue: implications for cell-based therapies. Tissue Eng. **7**, 211–228 (2001). https://doi.org/10.1089/107632701300062859
8. Neupane, M., Chang, C.C., Kiupel, M., Yuzbasiyan-Gurkan, V.: Isolation and characterization of canine adipose-derived mesenchymal stem cells. Tissue Eng. - Part A. **14**, 1007–1015 (2008). https://doi.org/10.1089/ten.tea.2007.0207
9. Dabrowska, S., Andrzejewska, A., Janowski, M., Lukomska, B.: Immunomodulatory and regenerative effects of mesenchymal stem cells and extracellular vesicles: therapeutic outlook for inflammatory and degenerative diseases. Front. Immunol. **11**, 591065 (2021). https://doi.org/10.3389/fimmu.2020.591065
10. Vieira, N.M., Brandalise, V., Zucconi, E., Secco, M., Strauss, B.E., Zatz, M.: Isolation, characterization, and differentiation potential of canine adipose-derived stem cells. Cell Transplant. **19**, 279–289 (2010). https://doi.org/10.3727/096368909X481764
11. Blecker, D., Elashry, M.I., Heimann, M., Wenisch, S., Arnhold, S.: New insights into the neural differentiation potential of canine adipose tissue-derived mesenchymal stem cells. J. Vet. Med. Ser. C Anat. Histol. Embryol. **46**, 304–315 (2017). https://doi.org/10.1111/ahe.12270
12. Prpar Mihevc, S., Kokondoska Grgich, V., Kopitar, A.N., Mohorič, L., Majdič, G.: Neural differentiation of canine mesenchymal stem cells/multipotent mesenchymal stromal cells. BMC Vet. Res. **16**, 1–12, 282 (2020). https://doi.org/10.1186/s12917-020-02493-2

13. Shah, K., et al.: Outcome of allogeneic adult stem cell therapy in dogs suffering from osteoarthritis and other joint defects. Stem Cells Int. **2018**, 7309201 (2018). https://doi.org/10.1155/2018/7309201
14. Kaur, G., et al.: A double-blinded placebo-controlled evaluation of adipose-derived mesenchymal stem cells in treatment of canine atopic dermatitis. Vet. Res. Commun. **46**(1), 251–260 (2021). https://doi.org/10.1007/s11259-021-09853-9
15. Falcão, M.S.A., et al.: Effect of allogeneic mesenchymal stem cells (MSCs) on corneal wound healing in dogs. J. Tradit. Complement. Med. **10**, 440–445 (2020). https://doi.org/10.1016/j.jtcme.2019.04.006
16. Bach, F.S., et al.: Comparison of the efficacy of surgical decompression alone and combined with canine adipose tissue-derived stem cell transplantation in dogs with acute thoracolumbar disk disease and spinal cord injury. Front. Vet. Sci. **6**, 1–11, 383 (2019). https://doi.org/10.3389/fvets.2019.00383
17. Pérez-Merino, E.M., et al.: Safety and efficacy of allogeneic adipose tissue-derived mesenchymal stem cells for treatment of dogs with inflammatory bowel disease: clinical and laboratory outcomes. Vet. J. **206**, 385–390 (2015). https://doi.org/10.1016/j.tvjl.2015.08.003
18. Yan, Y., et al.: Therapeutic applications of adipose-derived mesenchymal stem cells on acute liver injury in canines. Res. Vet. Sci. **126**, 233–239 (2019). https://doi.org/10.1016/j.rvsc.2019.09.004
19. Lee, K.S., et al.: Sequential sub-passage decreases the differentiation potential of canine adipose-derived mesenchymal stem cells. Res. Vet. Sci. **96**, 267–275 (2014). https://doi.org/10.1016/j.rvsc.2013.12.011
20. Requicha, J.F., Viegas, C.A., Albuquerque, C.M., Azevedo, J.M., Reis, R.L., Gomes, M.E.: Effect of anatomical origin and cell passage number on the stemness and osteogenic differentiation potential of canine adipose-derived stem cells. Stem Cell Rev. Reports. **8**, 1211–1222 (2012). https://doi.org/10.1007/s12015-012-9397-0
21. Screven, R., et al.: Immunophenotype and gene expression profile of mesenchymal stem cells derived from canine adipose tissue and bone marrow. Vet. Immunol. Immunopathol. **161**, 21–31 (2014). https://doi.org/10.1016/j.vetimm.2014.06.002
22. Lee, J., et al.: Effect of donor age on the proliferation and multipotency of canine adipose-derived mesenchymal stem cells. J. Vet. Sci. **18**, 141–148 (2017). https://doi.org/10.4142/jvs.2017.18.2.141
23. Zhao, Y., Waldman, S.D., Flynn, L.E.: The effect of serial passaging on the proliferation and differentiation of bovine adipose-derived stem cells. Cells Tissues Organs **195**, 414–427 (2012). https://doi.org/10.1159/000329254
24. Yang, Y.H.K., Ogando, C.R., Wang See, C., Chang, T.Y., Barabino, G.A.: Changes in phenotype and differentiation potential of human mesenchymal stem cells aging in vitro. Stem Cell Res. Ther. **9**, 1–14, 131 (2018). https://doi.org/10.1186/s13287-018-0876-3
25. Krešić, N., et al.: The expression pattern of surface markers in canine adipose-derived mesenchymal stem cells. Int. J. Mol. Sci. **22**, 7476 (2021). https://doi.org/10.3390/ijms22147476
26. Krešić, N., Šimić, I., Lojkić, I., Tomislav, B.: Canine adipose derived mesenchymal stem cells transcriptome composition alterations : a step towards standardizing therapeutic. Stem Cells Int. **2017**, 4176292 (2017). https://doi.org/10.1155/2017/4176292
27. Dominici, M., et al.: Minimal criteria for defining multipotent mesenchymal stromal cells. The International Society for Cellular Therapy position statement. Cytotherapy. **8**, 315–317 (2006). https://doi.org/10.1080/14653240600855905
28. Selle, M., et al.: Influence of age on stem cells depends on the sex of the bone marrow donor. J. Cell. Mol. Med. **26**, 1594–1605 (2022). https://doi.org/10.1111/jcmm.17201

29. Martinello, T., et al.: Canine adipose-derived-mesenchymal stem cells do not lose stem features after a long-term cryopreservation. Res. Vet. Sci. **91**, 18–24 (2011). https://doi.org/10.1016/j.rvsc.2010.07.024
30. Guercio, A., Di Bella, S., Casella, S., Marco, P.D., Russo, C., Piccione, G.: Canine mesenchymal stem cells (MSCs): characterization in relation to donor age and adipose tissue-harvesting site. Cell Biol. Int. **37**, 789–798 (2013). https://doi.org/10.1002/cbin.10090
31. Sasaki, A., et al.: Canine mesenchymal stem cells from synovium have a higher chondrogenic potential than those from infrapatellar fat pad, adipose tissue, and bone marrow. PLoS ONE **13**, 1–20, e0202922 (2018). https://doi.org/10.1371/journal.pone.0202922
32. Rashid, U., et al.: Characterization and differentiation potential of mesenchymal stem cells isolated from multiple canine adipose tissue sources. BMC Vet. Res. **17**, 1–12, 388 (2021). https://doi.org/10.1186/s12917-021-03100-8
33. Voga, M., Kovač, V., Majdic, G.: Comparison of canine and feline adipose-derived mesenchymal stem cells/medicinal signaling cells with regard to cell surface marker expression, viability, proliferation, and differentiation potential. Front. Vet. Sci. **7**, 1–13, 610240 (2021). https://doi.org/10.3389/fvets.2020.610240
34. Tan, K., et al.: CD73 expression on mesenchymal stem cells dictates the reparative properties via its anti-inflammatory activity. Stem Cells Int. **2019**, 8717694 (2019). https://doi.org/10.1155/2019/8717694
35. Takemitsu, H., Zhao, D., Yamamoto, I., Harada, Y., Michishita, M., Arai, T.: Comparison of bone marrow and adipose tissue-derived canine mesenchymal stem cells. BMC Vet. Res. **8**, 150 (2012). https://doi.org/10.1186/1746-6148-8-150
36. Davies, O.G., Cooper, P.R., Shelton, R.M., Smith, A.J., Scheven, B.A.: Isolation of adipose and bone marrow mesenchymal stem cells using CD29 and CD90 modifies their capacity for osteogenic and adipogenic differentiation. J. Tissue Eng. **6**, (2015). https://doi.org/10.1177/2041731415592356
37. James, J.L., et al.: The chondrogenic potential of first-trimester and term placental mesenchymal stem/stromal cells. Cartilage. **13**, 544–558 (2021). https://doi.org/10.1177/19476035211044822
38. Mikic, B., Ferreira, M.P., Battaglia, T.C., Hunziker, E.B.: Accelerated hypertrophic chondrocyte kinetics in GDF-7 deficient murine tibial growth plates. J. Orthop. Res. **26**, 986–990 (2008). https://doi.org/10.1002/jor.20574
39. Kumlin, M., Lindberg, K., Haldosen, L.-A., Felländer-Tsai, L., Li, Y.: Growth differentiation factor 7 promotes multiple-lineage differentiation in tenogenic cultures of mesenchymal stem cells. Injury **53**, 4165–4168 (2022). https://doi.org/10.1016/J.INJURY.2022.09.017
40. Tsuji-Tamura, K., Ogawa, M.: Morphology regulation in vascular endothelial cells. Inflamm. Regen. **38**, 1–13, 25 (2018). https://doi.org/10.1186/s41232-018-0083-8
41. Xu, X., Weinstein, M., Li, C., Deng, C.X.: Fibroblast growth factor receptors (FGFRs) and their roles in limb development. Cell Tissue Res. **296**, 33–43 (1999). https://doi.org/10.1007/s004410051264
42. Wang, J., et al.: Mechanical stimulation orchestrates the osteogenic differentiation of human bone marrow stromal cells by regulating HDAC1. Cell Death Dis. **7**, 1–12 (2016). https://doi.org/10.1038/cddis.2016.112
43. Lee, H.W., Suh, J.H., Kim, A.Y., Lee, Y.S., Park, S.Y., Kim, J.B.: Histone deacetylase 1-mediated histone modification regulates osteoblast differentiation. Mol. Endocrinol. **20**, 2432–2443 (2006). https://doi.org/10.1210/me.2006-0061
44. Li, J., et al.: TRAF4 positively regulates the osteogenic differentiation of mesenchymal stem cells by acting as an E3 ubiquitin ligase to degrade Smurf2. Cell Death Differ. **26**, 2652–2666 (2019). https://doi.org/10.1038/s41418-019-0328-3

45. Kolf, C.M., Cho, E., Tuan, R.S.: Mesenchymal stromal cells. Biology of adult mesenchymal stem cells: regulation of niche, self-renewal and differentiation. Arthritis Res. Ther. **9**, 1–10, 204 (2007). https://doi.org/10.1186/ar2116
46. Fink, T., et al.: Induction of adipocyte-like phenotype in human mesenchymal stem cells by hypoxia. Stem Cells. **22**, 1346–1355 (2004). https://doi.org/10.1634/stemcells.2004-0038
47. Haga, R.B., Ridley, A.J.: Rho GTPases: regulation and roles in cancer cell biology. Small GTPases. **7**, 207–221 (2016). https://doi.org/10.1080/21541248.2016.1232583

Brain Computer Interface in Neurology: The Future of Neurorestoration, the Possibilities and Perils. A Narrative Review

Slaven Lasić[1(✉)], Filip Đerke[1,2], Silvio Bašić[1,2], and Vida Demarin[3,4]

[1] Department of Neurology, Referral Centre for Preoperative Assessment of Patients With Pharmacoresistant Epilepsy, University Hospital Dubrava, Zagreb, Croatia
slasic@kbd.hr

[2] Department of Psychiatry and Neurology, Faculty of Dental Medicine and Health, JJ Strossmayer University of Osijek, Osijek, Croatia

[3] International Institute for Brain Health, Zagreb, Croatia

[4] Department of Medical Sciences, Croatian Academy of Sciences and Arts, Zagreb, Croatia

Abstract. Neurological diseases often leave a devastating effect on the quality of life of patients, and their caregivers. Usually, when people are healthy, communication and movement are taken for granted. Unfortunately when disease or trauma happens a disconnection from these basic aspects of life leaves a person stranded with current options still limited in alleviating these devastating situations. That is where Brain-Computer Interfaces come into play, as a novel way of replacing, and treating neurological diseases and injuries. Using advanced computer technologies direct brain activity can be used to issue commands through a computer or a replacement limb, wheelchair, or exoskeleton. Not only replacement but also neuromodulation and neurorehabilitation by way of BCI provide new ways of treating diseases with functional connectivity issues. More and more research is proving its usability, with awe-inspiring prospects for the future treatment of neurological diseases. But as with any technological novelty thorough discussion, and general informing of both the patients and clinicians is needed so as to prevent future worries and disappointment.

Keywords: Brain-Computer Interface · Neurorestoration · Neurorehabilitation · Narrative review

1 Brain – Computer Interface Introduction

Brain-computer interface (BCI) is a technological novelty with a slow pacing history usually associated with science fiction ideas of manipulating objects or computer applications with the thought of one's mind. It has been thought of and designed as a possible solution in assistive technology for the most severely disabled patients in neurology. Those who have lost almost all of the abilities of communication or movement are afflicted with severe diseases such as neuromuscular disease (amyotrophic lateral sclerosis, muscular dystrophies), cerebrovascular disease (stroke, locked–in syndrome),

P. Bonačić Bartolin et al. (Eds.): BioMedVetMech 2022, IFMBE Proceedings 90, pp. 19–34, 2024.
https://doi.org/10.1007/978-3-031-42243-0_2

traumatic injuries (spinal cord injury), cerebral palsy, and multiple sclerosis. First coined as "Brain-Computer Interface" by Jacques Vidal [1], its history dates back to the 1960s with research in different facets of potential uses rising exponentially from the 2010s to 2020s [2]. BCI uses the complex algorithmic decoders in distinguishing repeating previously singled-out features of neuronal electrical activity (or metabolic activity) and coupling it with the user's intent which is then translated, digitized, and transferred to a computer or a machine for command execution or neuromodulation. It serves as an artificial medium and a replacement in the central nervous system (CNS) – peripheral nervous system (PNS) axis replacing natural neurohumoral or neuromuscular output with an artificial one be it a machine (robotic hand, wheelchair) or computer (speech synthesizer, cursor control) [3]. BCI architecture comprises four essential components: signal acquisition, feature extraction, feature translation, and device output commands. Depending on their signal acquisition method BCIs are divided into invasive (which use microelectrode arrays, electrocorticorticogram (ECoG)) or noninvasive BCI (use primarily electroencephalogram (EEG), but also functional magnetic resonance imaging (fMRI), magnetoencephalography (MEG), functional near-infrared imaging (fNIRS)). BCI can be characterized as a dependent (need some form of PNS output like Vidal's gaze controlled BCI) or independent (BCI input is purely mental like motor imagery, no need for residual motor activity as in complete locked in syndrom), afferent (BCI output changes the brain thru neuromodulation, e.g. used in mood disorders) or efferent (BCI output is purely mechanical, e.g. wheelchair, robotic arm movement, speech synthesizer) [3].

1.1 Technical Aspects

Different methods for a signal acquisition offer various possibilities with EEG being primarily used due to its high temporal resolution (numbered in milliseconds), portability, and usability. Other methods such as microelectrode arrays (or ECoG to a lesser extent) use superb local micrometer spatial resolution and use direct action potentials of single neurons which are far superior in signal-to-noise ratio compared to spaced-out EEG signal being recorded on millions of neurons while being distorted with possible electromyography (EMG) artifacts of head muscle movement [3]. Invasive procedures also generate higher data bandwidth necessary for more complex movement or faster communication options. The superb local spatial resolution comes at a cost of surgical implantation reducing its usability and causing aversion to patients not inclined to surgical procedures [3, 4]. Other than signal acquisition, different types of signals are used to extract meaningful intent from the patient such as:

1. sensory-motor rhythms (SR) - the endogenous oscillatory activity of the thalamocortical network recorded over sensory-motor cortex whose changes in frequency amplitude can be learned to change and therefore convey the message
2. slow cortical potentials (SCP) - slow shifts in depolarization levels of pyramidal neurons occurring half a second after an internal event
3. event-related potentials (ERP) - time-fixed changes in EEG potentials associated with exogenous or endogenous events such as visual (VEP), steady-state visual (SSVEP), auditory (AEP), and tactile (TEP) related potentials

4. P300 event-related potentials – a large positive wave registered approximately 300 ms after a rarer form of two events unfolds triggering "oddball" event-related potential
5. spikes and local field potentials (LFP) – spikes present action potentials of singular neurons with information encoded in firing rates, local field potentials use synchronized events in neural populations recorded by microelectrode array (same principle only noninvasive is used by EEG)

Depending on the task a BCI is supposed to accomplish, different types of signals are used with sensory-motor rhythms using motor imagery to change sensory-motor oscillations causing the moving of objects, and P300 ERP is used mostly in letter selection in communication applications thru "row-column paradigm" and "oddball paradigm" [3, 5]. Motor imagery as a method requires time-consuming training of the user of BCI, while the "oddball paradigm" P300 mechanic is intuitive and thus time-saving, especially in patients who are unable to focus on BCI training and are mostly considered BCI illiterate [3, 5, 6]. Most of today's BCI use electrophysiological signals compared to metabolic ones (fMRI, MEG, fNIRS). This paper is going to focus mostly on electrophysiological BCI, for additional information regarding metabolic BCI the reader is referred to these papers [7, 8]. Decoding meaningful information from recorded brain wave activity requires a trained algorithm and decoder setup that uses one of the multiple classification techniques such as common spatial filter (CSF), wavelet transform (WT), Kalman filter (KF), linear discriminant analysis (LDA), support vector machine (SVM), and radial basis function (RBF). Combinations of signal processing and classifying methods offer various types of BCI and its function. Spatial, time and frequency domain filters can be used to discern usable signals to noise. The result in the translation process are continuous or discrete commands with continuous commands being dynamic real-time outcomes made by feeding the translational algorithm with small windowed signals (used for movement control e.g. prosthetic limb), and discrete commands being periodic fixed outcomes (e.g. letter selection). After all, is said and done mental intent of a subject is made in a command and then the outcome [9, 10].

1.2 Effects of BCI

CNS-PNS axis is a dynamic system with plasticity and adaptation during everyday physical and mental use being a form of maxim. Being that BCI represents a bypass of PNS so too it causes novel adaptation of the CNS to a new function with BCI adapting itself to the user's progress (or lack of one) using artificial intelligence, and neural networks to retrain itself. BCI's effect on brain plasticity is well documented with as little as one hour of BCI mental training in naive subjects causing discernible MRI changes in regions of the brain affected by a mental task [11]. If used correctly the possibilities of this technology in restorative and rehabilitative medicine are enormous. Today medicinal uses of this technology are only the beginning. A complex and somewhat too generalized form of BCI implementation in society poses other questions which need answering besides the best interest of patients suffering from neurological disease. That is why this review is essential, it is important to familiarise clinicians with this emerging technology, to show its positive sides, and discuss its far-reaching potentially altering effects on other aspects of society.

2 Implications in Neurology: Replacement, Restoration, and Neuromodulation

The usefulness of BCI in neurology reaches from enabling glimmers of communication with patients with consciousness disorders to replacing lost motor functions, treating movement disorders, recognizing and preventing seizures, or being part of a new rehabilitation paradigm for stroke.

2.1 Consciousness

BCI uses in the field of consciousness have opened new insights into the different stages of disorders of consciousness. Error rates of diagnosing vegetative state have been labeled to be as close to 40%, and now more than ever consciousness and its disturbances are being perceived as a dynamic condition as opposed to former rigid differentiation [12]. A report by Kulber and Kotchoubey poses a hierarchical theoretical option of proving possible ranges of consciousness in patients with disorders of consciousness (DOS) using a BCI system which can then conduct simple forms of communication using auditory and tactile stimulation-induced P300 [12]. They propose 4 step procedure that starts from recording rest EEG and auditory evoked potentials to exclude patients inadequate for BCI use, to passive stimulation, stimulation following instructions, volitional tasks (if patients perform above chance level, consciousness and cognitive processes can be indirectly inferred), and decision making with a BCI. On the same note, Muller-Putz et al. used simple MI by moving the left arm or right leg to encode yes or no binary answers in minimally conscious patients [13]. BCI offers a possibility to probe into the sea of consciousness a little further, giving the family of patients additional information in the decision-making process. Some patients in neurological intensive care unit (NeuroICU) have cognitive activity detected by fMRI but no outright behavioral output (termed cognitive motor dissociation CMD). A pilot study by Eliseyev et al. [14] proved that a self-paced BCI can be applied in an ICU environment as a form of communication with CMD patients, while their unconscious patients did not succeed in controlling the BCI. In their study, EEG signals of the intention of opening and closing the hand had been used to speed up or slow down an auditory signal which was used as a feedback signal. This application can offer relief for patients when suffering from discomfort, and in no way of signaling it.

2.2 Communication

Besides simpler forms of communication in patients suffering from DOS more advanced forms of communication with P300 and SSVEP BCI spellers have been studied and are going through clinical research with patients with a locked-in syndrome (LIS) or tetraplegia. Patients suffering from late-stage ALS, spinal cord injury, or LIS from stroke often have effortful, error-prone communication or no means of communication at all. For letter selection communication "row-column paradigm" has proven itself to be a valuable method with patients silently counting the number of flashes of the letter they wish to communicate amongst the other randomly flashed rows and columns of letters or numbers [15]. This method produces a P300 electrical activity in EEG after a wanted letter column, and afterward, rows are flashed enough times with a successful BCI communication rate of 77% and an estimated 17 bit/min of information transfer. Another P300 method checkerboard paradigm (CBD) advances some of the flaws of the row-column paradigm with better accuracy of 92% and more information being transferred at 23 bits/min [16]. The possibility of BCI communication has been proven in ALS patients with a 70% success rate reported in patients in a study group by Marchetti et al. [17]. Besides communication with BCI spellers, the quality of life of ALS patients can improve with free-form painting applications powered by BCI as presented in a study by Münßinger et al. [18]. Being that patients with advanced-stage of neuromuscular disorders such as ALS and genetic muscular dystrophies (Duchenne muscular dystrophy) suffer from attentional deficits a study by Utsumi et al. [19] designed a two-step region-based P300 BCI speller and tested it on patients with advanced stage Duchenne muscular dystrophy compared to able-bodied controls. They divided the letters into 6 regions each containing 9 letters. Analyzing a P300 signal the BCI was able to guess the target region, and afterward the letter, allowing the burden of attention to be divided between the BCI and the user. Accuracy in letter selection in patients was 71.6% (9.34 bit/min) which was comparable to 80,6% (11.24 bit/min) for able-bodied controls. Excellent work by F. R. Willet et al. [20] proved the spatial superiority of using a microelectrode array as it offered the possibility to decode engrained handwriting movement in the cortex of SCI tetraplegic subjects. They instructed their tetraplegic subject to attempt to write as if his hand was not paralyzed and to imagine he was using a pen to do so. Their study used a neural network decoder which reduced the time necessary to retrain the BCI, proved that handwriting notion is neurally represented years after the paralysis, and with a better spatiotemporal resolution of neural activity compared to the straight line used in point-to-point movements in point and click spellers. Their BCI accomplished astonishing typing speeds of 90 characters per minute with 94.1% raw online accuracy which compared to 1–5 characters per minute in BCI using oddball potentials, and 60 characters per minute with BCI using visual evoked potentials is the fastest BCI speller currently.

Most research done on patients using microelectrode array are technically demanding with cables connecting the BCI system directly with the scalp of the subject. A pilot study by J.D. Simeral et al. reports the first human use of broadband wireless intra-cortical BCI. The study was conducted on two tetraplegics SCI subjects whose neural spikes and LFPs were collected, and used to encode cursor control on a computer. This allowed the subject to freely type, use computer applications, and browse the internet without restraints. This study proved that there was similar accuracy between cabled and wireless BCI intracortical systems with a negligible increase in noise compared to signal. After resolving the technical issues of loss of signal, and deteriorating wireless signal quality (with space and objects between BCI electrodes and an antenna) potentially causing problems in more complex forms of output, wireless intracortical BCI have a potentially bright and fruitful future [21]. An interesting solution to invasive signal acquisition comes from a work by T.J. Oxley et al. [22] who used a minimally invasive stent electrode implanted over the sensory-motor cortex thru a venous catheter moved up to a superior sagittal sinus. They used the method of gathering different temporal patterns of electrophysiological signals associated with the intention of movement of upper or lower extremities to encode 3 types of commands, single click option, multiple click options, and zoom. They combined it with gaze-controlled steering of the cursor to enable two patients with upper limb ALS to communicate by typing, browsing the internet, managing online finance, and shopping. Their subjects achieved a click selection accuracy of 92.63%, and 93.18% respectively, with a rate of correct characters per minute of 13.81, and 20.10. This study proves that safe, previously known endovascular methods are making their way in a novel playing field such as BCI as well.

2.3 Movement

To elicit movement numerous parts of the CNS are needed for it to be calibrated and executed in a smooth and precise manner. Complex interactions between the primary motor cortex, supplementary motor cortex, prefrontal cortex, sensory cortex, subcortical structures (basal ganglia), cerebellum, lower motor neurons, and interneurons of the spinal cord are all responsible for executing an effortless and correct movement. It is by their grace that our movements are intuitive to our conscious experience. When a person suffers an SCI their spinal cord is disconnected from the rest of the CNS unable to receive instructions and commands to execute a movement. When a stroke patient suffers an injury of the primary motor cortex and or supplementary motor cortex, the whole sequence destabilizes and produces weak, inadequate movement (paresis), or is unable to produce any movement (plegia). Using the intact neuronal activity of the sensory-motor cortex in SCI patients in the form of mostly motor imagery, but also other forms of signal, movement intention can be decoded by the BCI and bypassing an injury conducted to a robotic arm or electrodes placed on the muscles of a paralyzed limb (functional electrical stimulation FES), wheelchair, or exoskeleton [9]. In stroke patients, ipsilesional leftover neurons of marginal movement fields (or contralesional) can be used as a signal area to elicit movement of the robotic limb, or FES-powered own limb to help in rehabilitation. Alongside communication, movement is a defining segment of self-image, and personhood, the lack of which affects the quality of life severely. Solving this issue helps patients in self-realisation, and helps lessen the burden on the caregivers.

Wheelchairs have been a backbone assistive appliance still requiring caregiver's effort or at least some leftover upper extremity strength to use. The possibility of controlling the movement of the wheelchair only using mental motor imagery is reported by J. Li et al. [23] in a study conducted on three healthy subjects. Their wheelchair system encoded directions and movement to mental motor imagery (left motor imagery to turn left, right motor imagery to turn right, feet motor imagery to go forward), and was free to use and move through space without a predetermined movement path. Upscaling the BCI-powered wheelchair paradigm by using multiple signals (MI, SSVEP, P300) simultaneously in wheelchair control allows multiple degrees of freedom of movement by way of direction, and speed as presented in a paper by J. Li et al. [24], and Y. Li et al. [25]. Besides using multi-signal options in controlling the BCI-powered wheelchair a study by J. Tang et al. [26] presents a BCI-controlled smart wheelchair system. Their system decodes the intentions of subjects from EEG P300 and EMG signal coupled with cameras, sensors, robotic arm, and artificial intelligence allowing subjects to confirm a target destination, and or object with the smart wheelchair system doing the proper planning and mapping of the movement and executing it. This system allows patients to issue small commands which then generate complex movements, shortening the time necessary to control the BCI.

Wheelchairs make way for a novel kind of replacement technology with BCI-powered robotic orthosis, and exoskeletons. Technical issues of long-term microelectrode signal acquisition, wireless transmission, trainability of a BCI, and four limb exoskeleton powered by mental imaging BCI have been tackled in a study by A. L. Benabid et al. [27]. In their study they implanted a long-term microelectrode array (over 2 years) in a tetraplegic subject suffering from cervical SCI, trained him and his BCI in a virtual environment by simulating the movement of an avatar, culminating in free use control of multiple degrees of movement and excellent walking control of a four limb exoskeleton. They proved that a microelectrode array can be implanted for several years and adequately used with minimal signal distortion, resolving issues of biocompatibility and shifting of the cortical area of interest. Their exoskeleton model is an ultimate method of movement assistive technology in patients afflicted by high SCI. Moving and grasping using a robotic arm with an average accuracy of 92.06% and an information transfer rate of 35.98 bits/min was reported in a study by Y. Zhu et al. [28] (Table 1). Their study used a hybrid BCI with SSVEP to issue commands to the robotic arm, and electrooculography detected eye blinks to start the SSVEP decoding command protocol. Even though their system requires less training time to be used, its visually intensive signal protocol is prone to inducing fatigue in subjects, while the necessity to have residual eye movement barres its potential use in patients with LCIS. A synonym used in conjunction with the meaning of BCI is a brain-machine interface (BMI). While both BCI and BMI imply the use of the neurophysiological potential of a brain of a subject to transfer command to a device (computer or mechanical device), a difference is made in a way that BMI in a more narrow sense is associated with movement assistive or replacement technologies such as robotic hands, exoskeletons or wheelchairs [10]. BCI/BMI-powered neuroprosthesis are making their way into clinical practice as FDA-approved devices. These are mostly dependent BCI/BMI meaning they need in some ways a functional PNS to deliver commands. Some of those devices are DEKA LUKE advanced prosthetic arm system (DARPA, VA) which uses EMG signals from remaining muscles to initiate multiple degrees of movement of a prosthetic arm, ReWalk exoskeleton (ARGO Medical Technologies), EKSO GT (Ekso Robotics) as a first exoskeleton approved for stroke patients, and Indego exoskeleton (Parker Hannifin) [29].

2.4 Neurorehabilitation

Almost half of all stroke patients end up in wheelchairs after the acute stage of stroke treatment has ended. Current rehabilitative strategies are more and more using virtual reality, and robotic orthoses alongside known physical therapy options [30, 31]. Unfortunately, almost all of those options are reserved for patients with mild or moderate paresis, while patients with plegia are usually rehabilitated with passive exercises conducted by physical therapists. The possibility of using mental imagination of movement to facilitate neuroplasticity of damaged neural pathways has been based on previous research which found that the same neurons associated with the movement are activated by the

Table 1. Overview of presented BCI research

Ref	Patient Group & Intervention	BCI signal acquisition	Outcome	Key results	Year of study
Communication					
Muller-Putz et al. [13]	10 Healthy volunteers, binary (yes/no) communication	EEG MI	1st session 4 above 70% accuracy, 2nd session 2 of 3 communicated yes/no above 90%	Weakly positive	2013
Eliseyev et al. [14]	18 ICU patients, and 5 healthy volunteers, self paced simple communication controlling beeping tone	EEG SR, visual and auditory feedback	All volunteers performed BCI task ($p < 0.001$), 5 of 14 conscious ICU patients performed BCI task, none of 4 unconscious patients	Mixed; Positive in conscious subjects, possibility of self paced BCI in ICU	2021
Marchetti et al. [17]	10 ALS patients, moving the computer cursor by covert visuospatial attention (VAO)	EEG ERP (P300 and LNC)	Accuracy of communication 70%, better performance with endogenous VAO	Positive	2013
Utsumi et al. [19]	8 bedridden patients with DMD, 8 able bodied controls, letter spelling	Two step EEG P300	Accuracy 71.6% (9.34 bit/min) comparable to 80.6% (11.24 bit/min) in controls	Positive	2018
F.R.Willet et al. [20]	1 tetraplegic subject, computer handwriting letter selection	Microelectrode array MI	94.1% online accuracy, 90 characters per minute typing speed	Positive, small sample	2021
T.J.Oxley et al. [22]	2 patients with ALS, communicating by computer typing, cursor control	Superior sagitall sinus stent electrode, EEG MI	Click accuracy of 92.63% and 93.18%, correct characters 13.81, and 20.10 per minute	Positive, small sample	2020

(*continued*)

Table 1. (*continued*)

Ref	Patient Group & Intervention	BCI signal acquisition	Outcome	Key results	Year of study
Movement					
J. Li et al. [23]	3 healthy volunteers, wheelchair control	EEG MI	Trial accuracy of 82.56%	Positive, small sample	2013
J. Tang et al. [26]	3 patients (stroke, SCI), and 4 healthy volunteers, smart wheelchair control	EEG P300 combined with YOLOv2 object detection system	All seven subjects completed all tests (success rate 100%)	Positive	2018
Y. Zhu et al. [28]	15 healthy volunteers, moving a robotic arm	Hybrid electrooculography and EEG SSVEP	Average accuracy 92.06%, information transfer rate 35.98 bits/min	Positive	2021
Neurorehabilitation					
A.A. Frolov et al. [34]	60 stroke patients, 42 in BCI group, 18 control sham group, robotic hand exoskeleton rehabilitation	EEG MI	Improvement in upper extremity motor function 30.1% in BCI group, 11.1% in control group	Weakly positive, RCT	2016
Mokienko et al. [36]	36 stroke patients, 16 in BCI group, 20 in control group, robotic hand exoskeleton rehabilitation	EEG MI	Significant improvement in motor hand function with BCI, no improvement in control group	Positive, RCT	2016

Abbreviations: Electroencephalogram EEG, motor imagery MI, sensory motor rhythm SR, intensive care unit ICU, event related potential ERP, late negative component LNC, Duchenne muscular dystrophy DMD, amyotrophic lateral sclerosis ALS, spinal cord injury SCI, steady state visual evoked potential SSVEP, randomized controlled trial - RCT

imagination, planning, and preparing of the movement [32–34]. This combined with the notion of Hebbian neuroplasticity by way of "neurons that fire together wire together" makes way for possible neurorehabilitation by way of using the leftover ipsilesional neurons in rehabilitating cortex areas damaged by stroke [35]. Using this knowledge combined with BCI-engaged movement of robotic orthosis or exoskeleton by way of kinesthetic feedback can create new rehabilitation options in patients with severe paresis and plegia. Most neurorehabilitative studies with BCI use motor imagery as a preferred mode because of logical spatial differentiation of a movement of different parts of the body already spread across the homunculus model of the sensory-motor cortex, and because MI BCI conveys better neuroplastic changes to the same parts of cortex from which they extract information. Motor imagery uses the idea of neurophysiological signals called event-related desynchronization (observation, preparation, and execution of movement induce a decrease of μ – and β – rhythm in the cortical area of an involved body part) and event-related synchronization (increase of μ – rhythm in regions of the brain representing body parts not involved with the task) to entrain those with an intent which is then conveyed to a device which executes the movement [34].

The technical problems of rehabilitative robotic exoskeleton movement in form of proportional derivative controller, working point trajectory and motor synergies are explored in a work by Frolov A.A. et al. [34]. Besides providing technical and theoretical information based on human and robotic movement in their paper they reported a blind randomized controlled study of a BCI-controlled robotic hand exoskeleton in neurorehabilitation of chronic stroke patients. Their study included 60 patients of which 42 were in the BCI group, and 18 were in the control sham group. The BCI group had an improvement in upper extremity motor function in 30.1% of patients, while the control group had an improvement in 11.1% of patients. Their study group reported improvement in hand motor function in all subgroups of deficit (mild, moderate, severe), with improvement in the pinch, and grasp functions of the paralyzed hand only in the BCI exoskeleton group. There was no age nor stroke duration effect on motor function recovery. They have presented the first active movement mode of rehabilitation for patients with plegia and severe paresis, with an overall 5 h of training per patient already reporting a positive effect. The notion that these are the first steps of a new rehabilitative paradigm is evident in the fact that in their study even though there were positive outcomes at multiple levels there was no statistically significant difference between BCI and control groups in the total evaluation of motor function recovery, with patients who used BCI reporting potential side effects in the form of fatigue, insomnia, depression necessitating potential future inquiry in side effects of BCI neurorehabilitation. Likewise, a study by Mokienko et al. [36] proves that chronic stroke patients have a sufficient quality of control of MI-based BCI in neurorehabilitative purposes with time after injury, extensivity of injury and localization of stroke injury not exhibiting effect on the quality of control of BCI. They divided 16 patients in the BCI group and 20 patients in the control group and found that statistically significant improvement in motor hand function was found in the BCI rehabilitation group compared to the control group. The best results were seen in patients in the early rehabilitation period (<6 months after injury). Three of their four BCI patients in the early rehabilitation period and one patient in the late rehabilitation period (>6 months up to 8 years) had a significant improvement of hand motor function in way of newly found ability to take objects in hand and to open a door knob. Even though studies propose a positive future for the BCI controlled exoskeleton hand rehabilitation in stroke a first systemic review on this topic by Baniqued et al. [37] shows that there is an unmet need for a standardized protocol in performing BCI research, additional engineering solutions are needed as to lessen the time wasted for BCI training, and propose that mental fatigue during rehabilitation process could be solved by way of gamifying the process and making it more entertaining.

2.5 Neuromodulation

Previous BCI systems were mostly efferent with an outcome being a manipulation of an outside object. Currently more and more BCI is finding its way into neuromodulation, and a new paradigm of "brain-computer–brain interface (BCBI)" is rising. Using the neurofeedback theory patients can modulate their brain activity by way of interacting with their preprocessed and visually represented digitized brain wave activity. This method is used in treating disorders of functional connectivity such as ADHD, anxiety, autism, movement disorders, and cognitive disorders. Other forms of neuromodulation come from closed-loop systems such as closed-loop deep brain stimulation using BCBI in Parkinson's disease, or closed-loop BCBI in treating epilepsy. These systems use electrodes previously used in invasive treatment (DBS in Parkinson's disease) or diagnostics (ECoG in epilepsy) coupled to a computer which recognizes pathological oscillations in neurons and then issues an electric pulse that stops the pathological signal and restores physiological neuronal activity [3, 38, 39].

A review by Laura Carelli et al. [39] explores the idea of BCI cognitive assessment and rehabilitation options. Their report shows research indicating that a BCI can be used to conduct a battery of cognitive testing in patients with minimal residual or no residual motor function. P300-powered BCI is considered a better option in cognitive testing of patients who alongside motor difficulties often have attention disorders, with SSVEP and P300-powered hybrid BCI successfully used in cognitive testing in patients with disorders of consciousness. The necessity to adjust traditional paper cognitive tests to BCI ones leads to difficulties making the BCI cognitive tests harder to compare to standardized original tests. With BCI cognitive testing mostly focused on patients with no residual motor function, BCI cognitive rehabilitation in various forms (memory, attention, behavioral modulation) has been explored in a more diverse setting with positive effects reported in patients with cognitive disorders, ADHD, autism spectrum, and even healthy elderly. Even though these BCI techniques show positive effects while still being in nascent form the durability of their positive effect, the potential need for frequent usage and long-term side effects still need additional research. The problem of cognitive BCI research compared to motor BCI is that higher cognitive functions are made possible by higher level interaction of spatially different parts of the cortex, and they are not feasibly tested on animal models compared to functions of movement. Previous research has had problems in defining the best possible control signals to use when testing memory encoding, and the best cortex localization from which to acquire signals. A study by Buch V.P. et al. tried to resolve this problem with the proposed network model of cognitive BCI used in their study. They used properties of functional and structural connectivity across the cortex to divide different brain regions in neural network nodes and then analyze their subsequent strength of connection based on phase locking or phase synchrony (regions that have synchronized frequencies during a cognitive task) as a control signal. Conducted on one subject who had stereotactically placed intracranial EEG or sEEG (as part of epilepsy monitoring) they proved that this form of global neural connectivity strength can accurately predict optimal cognitive performance [40]. Their model proposes a technically simple, easy-to-use global control signal in cognitive BCI evaluation which would be extremely useful in future cognitive rehabilitation if only confirmed on a larger number of subjects.

Potential neuromodulatory BCI uses in pharmacoresistant epilepsy are presented in a paper by Rafeed Alkawadri. It reports that the untapped potential of a real-time recording made by intracranial EEG can be used to predict seizure onset in real-time by way of superior computing of BCI powered by machine learning, and artificial neural networks, and react upon it preventing its manifestation. Novel ways of defining functional connectivity, and oscillations in the epileptogenic zone and their usage in BCI are also discussed [41].

Recent research appreciates focal dystonias more and more as being a neural network disorder involving not only subcortical structures (basal ganglia, thalamus, and cerebellum) but also premotor, and parietal cortical regions with structural and functional disorganization leading to debilitating movements. This approach to the pathophysiology of dystonias gives an opening to potential BCI neuromodulation of functional connectivity. A study by K Simonyan et al. explores the idea of BCI use in treating a model patient with task-specific focal dystonia (laryngeal dystonia) by using an EEG-recorded signal over the premotor and parietal cortex [42]. They propose that a BCI can interpret an EEG recording of pathological brain activity during a dystonia-prevented speech, and visually present it in contrast to an EEG recording of physiological brain activity during an unaffected normal whisper. With this visual feedback, a patient could potentially modulate a disordered brain signal and try to stabilize it so it comes as close to a normal brain signal during an unobstructed whisper. This theory gives a new non-invasive way of treating focal dystonia patients. It still needs thorough clinical tests to see how often the patient needs to perform this type of treatment for an effect, how long does the effect last, what side effects will sprout, and whether will they be enough to preclude further treatment.

3 Ethical Implications of BCI Use

BCI as a technological solution to numerous life-shattering neurological disease states is mostly welcomed with open hands by patients and their caregivers. Sometimes these opinions are grounded in unrealistic optimism and high expectations. Therefore it is important to acknowledge the potential shortcomings of this technology. Discussions concerning ethical issues, issues concerning safety, and the overall holistic well-being of users are needed. Examples of ethical issues stumbled upon during the BCI research are discussed in a paper by P. McCullagh et al. [43]. Questions are numerous, and thorough debate is needed. What happens when a NeuroICU LIS patient gains a newfound meaning to communicate and acknowledge his/hers current state? Who's right it is to impose that potentially devastating knowledge on a person who could have been in a state of blissful ignorance? What happens when a BCI system fails, is it a fault of the patient or a technical issue? What effect will that have on a patient knowing that even the new technology cannot resolve his/hers issue? What happens when a patient gains a new potential output with the successful application of a BCI in clinical research only to be stripped of it needing to wait for years for that same BCI to properly develop? Some of the answers to these questions are proposed in the same work by P. McCullagh such as: creating an ethical advisory board during the clinical trials, and the making of the BCI, making BCI less technically demanding while more reliable, detailed screening of potential BCI user, informing the patient and all included about the positive possibilities, potential failure, and boundaries of success of a BCI. As previously discussed BCI could be used in multiple ways, but as with any treatment it too has to follow the tenets of medicine. The complexity of BCI usage in medicine stems from the fact that BCI blurs the lines between certain facts such as treatment and enhancement, between biological, and artificial, and between consciously intentional, and potentially changed by machine learning decoder. If used in neuromodulation who is the one governing the parameters for effective treatment for i.e. depression, ADHD, or cognitive disorder? What is considered to be healthy, and what is considered to be a marker of disease? If a person using a BCI for communication has a subclinical sign of dementia detected by BCI how to proceed with that knowledge? BCI such as other medical devices provides alleviation, and replacement of lost functions, but not the cure. But the effect a BCI can have on a person is on an unprecedented scale, with changes in the perception of self-being a reality not encountered previously [44].

With the blurring of the lines between treatment, and enhancement sooner or later BCI will transfer from the clinical domain to the public arena. Already companies such as Neuralink are enhancing the technical properties of a BMI system with the future possibility of using an intracortical BMI for clinical and commercial enhancement properties [45]. Companies such as EMOTIV are commercializing non-invasive EEG BCI for purposes such as citizen research, gaming, and hand-free control systems. If it comes to the enhancement use of BCI the prospect of a BCI-enhanced competition will persuade persons not inclined to it to accommodate to a more demanding sociological phenomenon. The dangers of that phenomenon are excellently discussed in the work by S. Lesaja and X. L. Palmer titled "Brain-Computer Interfaces and the Dangers of Neurocapitalism" [46]. Besides corporate, and authoritarian uses individuals with malicious intent can use the BCI to directly extract private information from patients or persons using it. Terms such as "neurocrime", and "brain hacking" prove that these ideas have permeated social consciousness and their implications are discussed in a paper by M. Ienca and P. Haselager [47].

4 Conclussion

Even though the grand-scale use of BCI in medicine and society at large is still in the not-so-far but not so near future the number of ongoing trials, and papers published shows that the progress, and interest of scientists, clinicians, patients, and the general public is exponentially rising. The possibility to resolve paralysis, communicate with loved ones, to predict and modulate disease in real time is astonishing, and awe-inspiring. The future of BCI looks promising only if the process of creation and use is transparent and if the medical and general public is informed and up to date. However if left unchecked both technical, and ethical issues can lead to skepticism at best, and patient harm at worst. The future is coming, and it is up to us to decide which way we want to go.

References

1. Vidal, J.J.: Toward direct brain – computer communication. Annu. Rev. Biophys. Bioeng. **2**(1), 157–180 (1973)
2. Li, C., Zhao, W.: Progress in the brain – computer interface: an interview with Bin He. Natl. Sci. Rev. **7**, 480–483 (2020)
3. He, B., Yuan, H., Meng, J., Gao, S.: Brain – computer interfaces. In: He, B. (eds): Neural engineering. Third edition, pp. 131–183. Springer Nature, Cham, Switzerland (2020)
4. Akinin, A., Akshkay, P., Wang, J., Buccino, A., Cauwenberghs, G.: Biopotential measurements and electrodes. In: He, B. (eds.) Neural engineering. Third edition, p. 65–96. Springer Nature, Cham, Switzerland (2020)
5. Fazel-Rezai, R., Allison, B.Z., Guger, C., Sellers, E.W., Kleih, S.C., Kübler, A.: P300 brain computer interface: current challenges and emerging trends. Frontiers in Neuroengineering **5**, 1–14 (2012)
6. Minkyu, A., Sung, C.J.: Performance variation in motor imagery brain–computer interface: a brief review. J. Neurosci. Methods **243**, 103–110 (2015)
7. Naseer, N., Hong, K.-S.: fNIRS – based brain – computer interfaces: a review. Front. Hum. Neurosci. **9**(3), 1–14 (2015)
8. Weiskopf, N., et al.: Principles of a brain – computer interface (bci) based on real – time functional magnetic resonance imaging (fMRI). IEEE Trans. Miodecial Eng. **51**(6), 966–970 (2004)
9. Burns, A., Adeli, H., Buford, A.J.: Brain-computer interface after nervous system injury. Neuroscientist **20**(6), 1–13 (2014)
10. Oby, R.E., Hennig, J.A., Batista, A.P., Yu, B.M., Chase, S.M.: Intracortical brain – machine interfaces. In: He, B. (eds). Neural engineering. Third edition, pp. 185–221. Springer Nature, Cham, Switzerland (2020)
11. Nierhaus, T., Vidaurre, C., Sannelli, C., Mueller, K.-R., Villringer, A.: Immediate brain plasticity after one hour of brain – computer interface (BCI). J Physiol **599**, 2435–2451 (2021)
12. Kübler, A., Kotchoubey, B.: Brain–computer interfaces in the continuum of consciousness. Curr Opin Neurol **20**(6), 643–649 (2007)
13. Müller-Putz, G.R., Pokorny, C., Klobassa, D.S., Horki, P.: A single-switch BCI based on passive and imagined movements: Toward restoring communication in minimally conscious patients. Int J Neural Syst **23**(2), 1250037
14. Eliseyev, A., et al.: Development of a brain-computer interface for patients in the critical care setting. PLoS ONE **16**(1), 1–13 (2021)
15. Farwell, L.A., Donchin, E.: Talking off the top of your head: toward a mental prosthesis utilizing eventrelated brain potentials. Electroencephalogr. Clin. Neurophysiol **70**(6), 510–523 (1988)
16. Townsend, G., et al.: A novel P300-based brain-computer interface stimulus presentation paradigm: moving beyond rows and columns. Clin. Neurophysiol. **121**(7), 1109–1120 (2010)
17. Marchetti, M., Piccione, F., Silvoni, S., Gamberini, L., Priftis, K.: Covert visuospatial attention orienting in a brain-computer inteface for amyotrophic lateral slerosis patients. Neurorehabil. Neural Repair **27**(5), 430–438 (2013)
18. Münßinger, J.I., et al.: Brain Painting: first evaluation of a new brain – computer interface application with ALS-patients and healthy volunteers. Front. Neurosci. **4**, 1–11 (2010)
19. Utsumi, K., Takano, K., Okahara, Y., Komori, T., Onodera, O., Kaansaku, K.: Operation of a P300-based brain-computer interface in patients with Duchenne muscular dystrophy. Sci Rep **8**, 1753 (2018)

20. Willet, F.R., Avansino, D.T., Hochberg, L.R., Henderson, J.M., Shenoy, K.V.: High-performance brain-to-text communication via handwriting. Nature **593**, 249–254 (2021)
21. Simeral, J.D., Hosman, T., Saab, J., Flesher, S.N., Vilela, M., Franco, B., et al.: Home use of a percutaneous wireless intracortical brain-computer interface by individuals with tetraplegia. IEEE Trans. Biomedical Eng. **68**(7), 2313–2325 (2021)
22. Oxley, T.J., Yoo, P.E., Rind, G.S., Ronayne, S.M., Lee, C.M.S., Bird, C., et al.: Motor neuroprosthesis implanted with neurointerventional surgery improves capacity for activities of daily living tasks in severe paralysis: first in-human experience. J. NeuroInterventional Surgery **13**(2), 102–108 (2020)
23. Li, J., Liang, J., Zhao, Q., Li, J., Hong, K., Zhang, L.: Design of assistive wheelchair system directly steered by human thoughts. Int. J. Neural Syst. **23**(3), 1350013 (2013)
24. Li, J., et al.: Evaluation and application of a hybrid brain computer interface for real wheelchair parallel control with multi-degree of freedom. Int. J. Neural Syst. **24**(4), 1450014 (2014)
25. Li, Y., Pan, J., Wang, F., Zhuliang, Y.: A hybrid BCI system combining P300 and SSVEP and its application to wheelchair control. IEEE Trans. Biomed. Eng. **60**(11), 3156–3166 (2013)
26. Tang, J., Liu, Y., Hu, D., Zhou, Z.: Towards BCI-actuated smart wheelchair system. Biomed. Eng. Online **17**, 1–22 (2018)
27. Benabid, A.L., Costecalde, T., Eliseyev, A., Charvet G., Verney, A., Karakas, S., et al.: An exoskeleton controlled by an apidural wireless brain-machine interface in a tetraplegic patient: a proof-of-concept demonstration. Lancet Neurol **18**(12), 1112–1122 (2019)
28. Zhu, Y., Li, Y., Lu, J., Li, P.: A hybrid BCI based on SSVEP and EOG for robotic arm control. Front. Neurorobot. **14**, 583641 (2020)
29. Young, M.J., Lin, D.J., Hochberg, L.R.: Brain-computer interfaces in neurorecovery and neurorehabilitation. Semin Neurol **41**(02), 206–216 (2021)
30. Garro, F., Chiappalone, M., Bucelli, S., De Michieli, L., Semprini, M.: Neuromechanical biomarkers for robotic neurorehabilitation. Front Neurorobot. **15**, 742163 (2021)
31. Lo, A.C., Guarino, P., Krebs, H.I., Volpe, B.T., Bever, C.T., Duncan, P.W., et al.: Multicenter randomized trial of robot-assisted rehabilitation for chronic stroke: methods and entry characteristics for VA ROBOTICS. Neurorehabil. Neural Repair **23**(8), 775–783 (2009)
32. Frolov, A.A., Husek, D., Silchenko, A.,V., Tintera, J., Rydlo, J.: The changes in the hemodynamic activity of the brain during motor imagery training with the use of brain-computer interface. Human Physiology **42**, 1–12 (2016)
33. Jeannerod, M.: The representing brain: neural correlates of motor intention and imagery. Behavioral and Brain Sci. **17**(2), 187–202 (1994)
34. Frolov, A.A., Húsek, D. , Biryukova, E.V., Bobrov, P.D., Mokienko, O.A., Alexandrov, A.V.: Principles of motor recovery in post-stroke patients using hand exoskeleton controlled by the brain-computer interface based on motor imagery. Neural Network World **27**(1), 107–137 (2017)
35. Hebb, D.O.: The Organization of Behavior. Wiley, New York USA (1949)
36. Mokienko, O.A., Lyukmanov, R.K., Chernikova, L.A., Suponeva, N.A., Piradov, M.A., Frolov, A.A.: Brain-computer interface: the first experience of clinical use in Russia. Human Physiology **42**(1), 24–31 (2016)
37. Baniqued P.D.E., Stanyer, E.C., Awais, M., Alazmani, A., Jackson, A.E., Mon-Williams, M.A. et al.: Brain-computer interface robotics for hand rehabilitation after stroke: a systemic review. J NeuroEngineering Rehabil **18**(15), 1–25 (2021)
38. Gunduz, A.: Deep brain stimulation: emerging technologies and applications. In: He, B. (eds.) Neural engineering. Third edition, pp. 223–243. Springer Nature, Cham, Switzerland (2020)
39. Carelli, L., Solca, F., Faini, A., Meriggi, P., Sangalli, D., Cipresso, P., et al.: Brain-computer interface for clinical purposes: cognitive assessment and rehabilitation. Biomed. Res. Int. **2017**(1695290), 1–11 (2017)

40. Buch, V.P., Richardson, A.G., Brandon, C., Stiso, J., Khattak, M.N., Basset, D.S. et al.: Nerwork brain-computer interface (nBCI): an alterrnative approach for cognitive prosthetics. Frontiers in Neuroscience **12**, 1–9 (2018)
41. Alkawadri, R.: Brain-computer interface (BCI) applications in mapping of epileptic brain networks based on intracranial-EEG: an update. Front. Neurosci **13**, 1–13 (2019)
42. Simonyan, K., Ehrlich, S.K., Andersen, R., Brumberg, J., Guenther, F., Hallet, M., et al.: Brain-computer interfaces for treatment of focal dystonia. Mov. Disord. **37**(9), 1798–1802 (2022)
43. McCullagh, P., Lightbody, G., Zygierewicz, J., Kernohan, W.G.: Ethical challenges associated with the development and deployment of brain computer interface technology. Neuroethics **7**(2), 109–122 (2013)
44. Klein, E.: Ethics and the emergence of brain-computer interface medicine. In: Ramsey, N.F., Millán, J.R. (eds). Handbook of clinical neurology, **168**, pp. 329–339, Elsevier (2020)
45. Musk, E.: An integrated brain-machine interface platform with thousands of channels. J Med Internet Res **22**(10), e16194 (2019)
46. Lesaja, S., Palmer, X.L.: Brain-Computer Interfaces and the Dangers of Neurocapitalism. arXiv preprint 2009.07951, pp. 1–15 (2020)
47. Ienca, M., Haselager, P.: Hacking the brain: brain-computer interfacing technology and the ethics of neurosecurity. Ethics Inf. Technol. **18**(2), 117–129 (2016)

High Wall Shear Stress and Its Gradient Indicates Intimal Hyperplasia in Vascular Bypass Graft End-to-Side Distal Anastomosis

Severino Krizmanić[1](✉), Dino Papeš[2], Predrag Pavić[2], and Zdravko Virag[1]

[1] Faculty of Mechanical Engineering, Department of Fluid Mechanics, University of Zagreb, I. Lučića 5, 10000 Zagreb, Croatia
severino.krizmanic@fsb.hr

[2] Department of Surgery, University of Zagreb, University Hospital Center Zagreb, Kišpatićeva 12, 10000 Zagreb, Croatia

Abstract. Simulation of three-dimensional (3D) blood flow in a distal end-to-side anastomosis for two total graft flowrate redistributions was performed. For the same total blood flow, the distal end-to-end anastomosis was analyzed. The aim was to analyze the applicability of two hypotheses for intimal hyperplasia (IH) formation in a distal anastomosis of bypass graft: (i) high WSS combined with high WSS gradient and (ii) low wall shear stress (WSS) combined with high stress oscillations. A newly proposed endothelial stretching index (ESI), related to the first hypothesis, and the Relative retention time (RRT), related to the second hypothesis, were calculated over the graft and artery wall, and compared in the considered cases. High ESI regions within end-to-side distal anastomosis correlate very well with regions that were observed to develop IH in vivo. In such anastomosis, the stagnation point in the velocity field travels significantly along the artery floor within a heart period, resulting with highly oscillatory wall shear stress and its high gradient, and predisposing for the IH formation. In end-to-end anastomosis, the obtained values of these two indices are low, which correlates well with low predisposition for IH formation in this type of anastomosis. In the region close to the suture line the high value of ESI indicates IH formation, offering an additional explanation for IH initiation. When planning surgery, it is better to choose an end-to-end distal anastomosis configuration when possible. One possible solution for reducing IH in the end-to-side distal anastomosis is replacing the part of the native artery subjected to high-oscillatory wall shear stress with a prefabricated prosthetic graft.

Keywords: Wall Shear Stress · Oscillatory Wall Shear Stress Index · Relative Retention Time · Wall Shear Stress Gradient · Endothelial Stretching Index

1 Introduction

The number of lower extremity revascularization procedures is increasing due to ageing of the population and will to active lifestyle and mobility. In the case of critically ischemic lower extremity the open bypass is the best solution [1]. When a lower extremity bypass

P. Bonačić Bartolin et al. (Eds.): BioMedVetMech 2022, IFMBE Proceedings 90, pp. 35–45, 2024.
https://doi.org/10.1007/978-3-031-42243-0_3

procedure is performed, either autologous saphenous vein or prosthetic vascular grafts are anastomosed end-to-side both proximally and distally. Although the vein offers superior long-term patency, especially for below-the-knee procedures, it is often unavailable or of insufficient quality. The end-to-side distal anastomosis is usually chosen to ensure blood supply both caudally and cranially from the distal anastomosis (Fig. 1). A significant problem with such configuration is graft thrombosis, which almost exclusively occurs at the distal anastomotic site. The major factor is intimal hyperplasia, caused by intimal and sub-intimal cell proliferation that eventually lead to anastomotic narrowing, turbulent flow, and thrombosis, after the neointimal plaque grows to a certain critical point. Intimal hyperplasia is the main cause of re-stenosis and graft failure after vascular reconstruction of small diameter blood vessels (diameter 2–6 mm) [2]. Intimal hyperplasia on the end-to-side anastomosis is seen at the anastomotic heel, toe, and arterial floor (Fig. 1). While intimal hyperplasia in toe and heel may be caused, among others, by reaction to foreign body (prosthetic graft and sutures) in the floor region it is mainly caused by blood stream shearing the intimal layer.

Intimal hyperplasia is caused by an inflammatory reaction due to mechanical stimulation or damage to the intimal cells. This leads to the accumulation of fibroblast and smooth muscle cell in the intima with extracellular matrix (ECM) deposition. It is a complex processes of cell proliferation, cell migration and ECM deposition and it involves multiple growth factors (PDGF, EGF and FGF), inflammatory cytokines (IL-6 and IL-8) and interaction of various cells (endothelial cells, SMCs, macrophages, and platelets). The finding of large numbers of inflammatory and giant cells in neo-intimal layers, and high local levels of inflammatory markers have been confirmed in multiple biochemical and histological studies [3].

There is a strong correlation between the formation of intimal hyperplasia and hemodynamic parameters: wall shear stress (WSS) magnitude, WSS oscillations, and WSS spatial gradient (WSSg) [4, 5]. Direct measurement of these parameters in a real vascular system is a difficult task and can only be performed at a limited number of points. Therefore, Computational Fluid Dynamics (CFD) is used, which provides information on velocity, pressure and viscous forces at millions of points and calculation of various parameters is simple. However, experimental measurements are crucial in the verification of computational results.

In vitro experiments [6] were performed in a specially designed flow chambers to examine the effect of positive and negative WSSg along with high WSS on bovine aortic endothelial cells (previously cultured at chamber walls). Authors observed that the high WSS/high positive WSSg combination had a negative impact on EC function, whereas high WSS/negative WSSg did not. Also, the condition of low WSS combined with the high WSS oscillation [7] may have a negative impact on the arterial wall. Based on the literature review two leading hypotheses are proposed [8]:

Hypothesis (a): High WSS and positive WSSg cause EC damage, extracellular matrix (ECM) degradation, and mural cell apoptosis.

Hypothesis (b): Low WSS and highly oscillatory WSS cause inflammatory effects on ECs, infiltration of inflammatory cells, proliferation and migration of smooth muscle cells, and thrombus formation.

Both hypotheses are important for defining pathways of intracranial aneurysm growth and rupture.

Here, the two hypotheses were checked in the case of IH in distal end-to-end anastomosis. The aims of this initial study are to:

1) create a CFD model for calculating blood flow and wall shear stress analysis at the distal prosthetic graft-native artery anastomosis,
2) define and calculate indices identifying regions of low WSS/highly oscillatory WSS and high WSS/high-positive WSSg, and to verify if the regions correspond to commonly in vivo observed IH regions,
3) propose a possible solution to reduce IH in distal end-to-side anastomosis.

2 Materials and Methods

OpenFoam software library [9] was used to simulate 3D flow in a bypass configuration, schematically shown in Fig. 1. In the distal anastomosis, the total blood flow Q_{tot} is divided into Q_d towards periphery and Q_p in backward direction towards blockage. We analyzed two cases: (A) $Q_d = 0.8Q_{\text{tot}}$; $Q_p = 0.2Q_{\text{tot}}$ (when the bypass graft delivers blood in both direction) and (B) $Q_d = Q_{\text{tot}}$; $Q_p = 0$ (when blood flows towards periphery only). In addition, we analyzed the end-to end bypass configuration in which the graft is directly connected to the distal artery (case C).

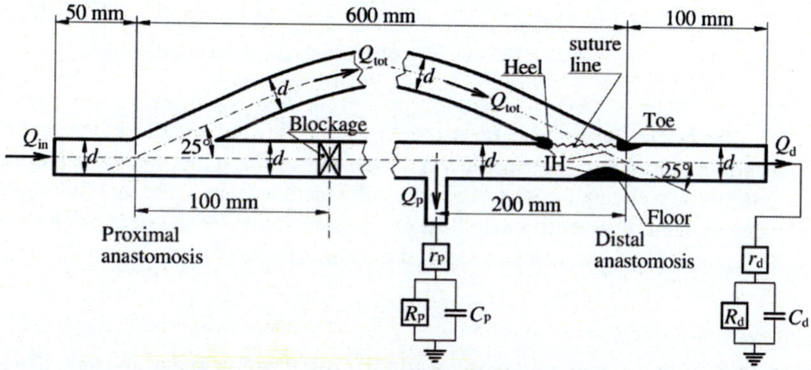

Fig. 1. Schematic view of the computational domain and outlet boundary conditions.

We made the following assumption: (1) the artery and graft had the same and constant diameter $d = 7$ mm, and their walls were rigid; (2) blood is a Newtonian fluid of constant density $\rho = 1060$ kg/m^3 and viscosity $\mu = 3{,}5$ mPa $\cdot$ s; (3) blood flow is laminar; and (4) impact of gravity is negligible.

At the inlet a time varying volume flowrate is prescribed (Fig. 2) assuming the flat velocity profile. At outlets, the pressure-volume flow rate relationship is defined by the three-element Windkessel model [10], which is presented in Fig. 1 in form of an electrical analogue scheme, where R is the peripheral resistance, C is the compliance, and r is the characteristic impedance of the resting part of the vascular system. At both outlets we assume $(R+r)C = 1$ s and $r/R = 0.064$. Distal and proximal peripheral resistances in the case (A) were $R_d = 78.2$ mmHg · s/ml and $R_p = 312.7$ mmHg · s/ml, respectively, while in cases (B) and (C) $R_d = 31.3$ mmHg · s/ml and $R_p = 10^{30}$ mmHg · s/ml. . The computational domain was divided into 1.1725 million finite volumes (a grid independence study was also performed).

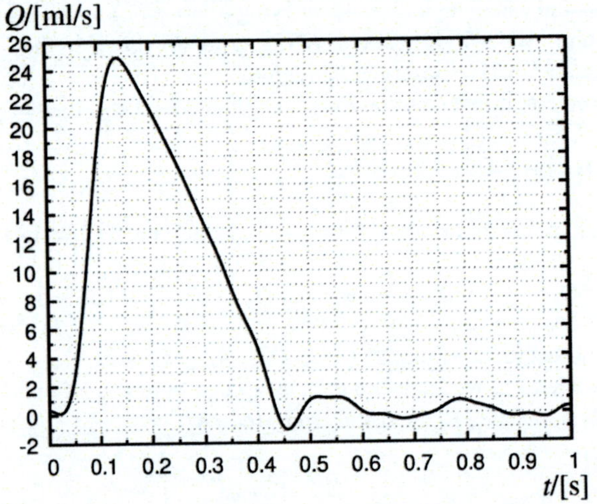

Fig. 2. Time varying blood flowrate at the domain inlet.

The Navier-Stokes equations were integrated by the time step of $\Delta t = 0.1$ ms over 6 heart periods (sufficient to achieve a steady state cyclic solution), and the results from the last period were analyzed. Obtained results included: the scalar pressure field p, vector velocity field $\vec{v}$ and the tensor field of viscous stresses τ. The vector of wall shear stress (tangential force per unit surface of the wall) is defined as:

$$\vec{\tau}_w = \vec{n} \cdot \tau - (\vec{n} \cdot \tau \cdot \vec{n})\vec{n} \tag{1}$$

where $\vec{n}$ is unit normal to the wall, and dot denotes scalar product. Time averaged magnitude of this vector $\tau_w = |\vec{\tau}_w|$ is called the wall shear stress (WSS) and when divided by the blood viscosity it is called wall shear rate [4] (WSR = WSS/μ). Besides WSS, both oscillatory shear index [11] (OSI) and wall shear stress gradient (WSSg) play an important role in formation of IH. The OSI is defined as:

$$\text{OSI} = \frac{1}{2}\left(1 - \frac{\left|\int_0^T \vec{\tau}_w dt\right|}{\int_0^T |\vec{\tau}_w| dt}\right) \tag{2}$$

where T is the heart period. The OSI is zero valued when components of $\vec{\tau}_w$ do not change sign, and its maximum value is 0.5.The vector of WSSg (here defined as space derivation of $\vec{\tau}_w$ in the direction of $\vec{\tau}_w$) is in a 3D flow defined as:

$$\overrightarrow{\mathrm{WSSg}} = \frac{\vec{\tau}_w}{|\vec{\tau}_w|} \cdot [\nabla \vec{\tau}_w] \tag{3}$$

where ∇ is the del operator, and the dot denotes the scalar product.

For identification of regions of small WSS and high OSI, related to Hypothesis (b) defined in Introduction, the relative retention time (RRT) is defined [12] as:

$$\mathrm{RRT} = [(1 - 2 \cdot \mathrm{OSI}) \cdot \mathrm{WSR}]^{-1} \tag{4}$$

For identification of regions of high WSS and high positive WSSg (directional derivation of $\vec{\tau}_w$ in direction of $\vec{\tau}_w$ defining the force that augments stretching of ECs), we define a new parameter ESI (Endothelial Stretching Index) as the time average of the following scalar product:

$$\mathrm{ESI} = \frac{1}{T} \int_0^T \left(\vec{\tau}_w \cdot \overrightarrow{\mathrm{WSSg}} \right) dt \tag{5}$$

which takes high values in case of high WSS and/or high WSSg, indicating possible incidence of IH according to the Hypothesis (a).

3 Results

Figures 3, 4 and 5 show the results for ESI and RRT indices calculated in the three cases. The top panel in each figure shows the distribution of ESI parameter at the half of the arterial wall (on the other half the distribution is symmetric), middle panel shows the same for RRT, and the bottom panel shows the line distribution of ESI and RRT along the artery floor.

4 Discussion

Although currently no threshold critical value of the newly proposed index ESI exists, artery floor values from the case of end-to-end anastomosis can be taken as a reference (in Fig. 5 the ESI values at artery floor are less than 500 Pa^2/m). For coloring of ESI surface distribution, we use thresholds: 500 and 1500 Pa^2/m. Values between these thresholds we considered high, and above 1500 Pa^2/m as extremely high, and both could be considered indicative for IH formation.

The RRT thresholds were set based on previous research [13] in which the HOLMES index was defined as: HOLMES $=$ WSS $\cdot$ (0.5 $-$ OSI), and which relates to RRT by the following equation:

$$\mathrm{RTT} = \frac{\mu}{2 \cdot \mathrm{HOLMES}} \tag{6}$$

Authors concluded that low HOLMES values (HOLMES < 0.5 Pa or RRT > 0.035 s) predict the incidence of IH better than WSS or OSI alone. Based on this, we defined

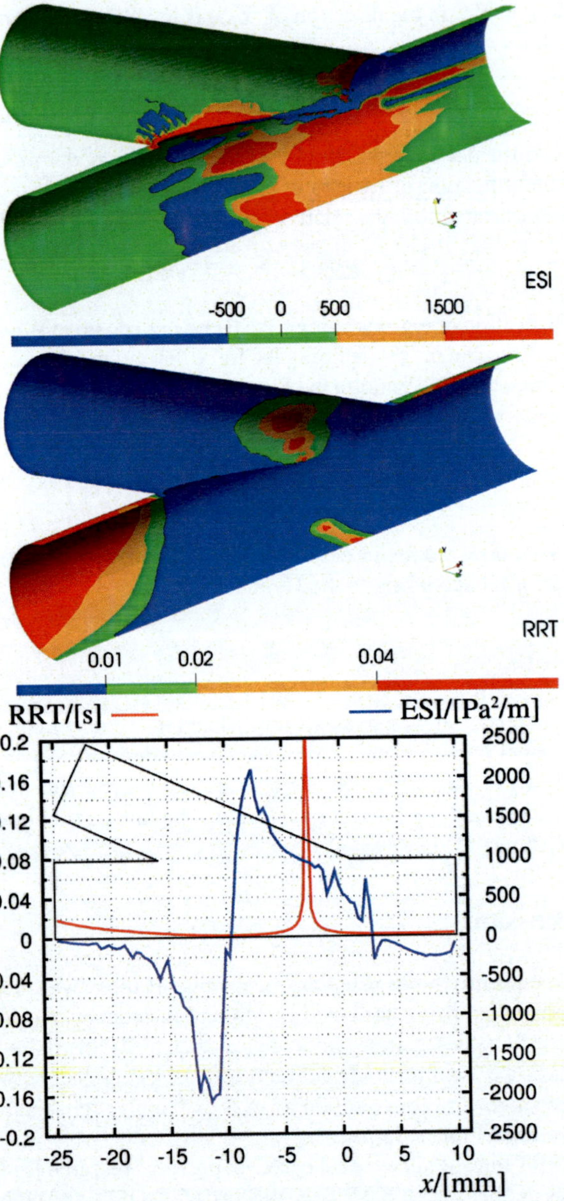

Fig. 3. Results for case (A): end-to-side distal anastomosis with the arterial blood flow in both caudal (80%) and cranial (20%) direction.

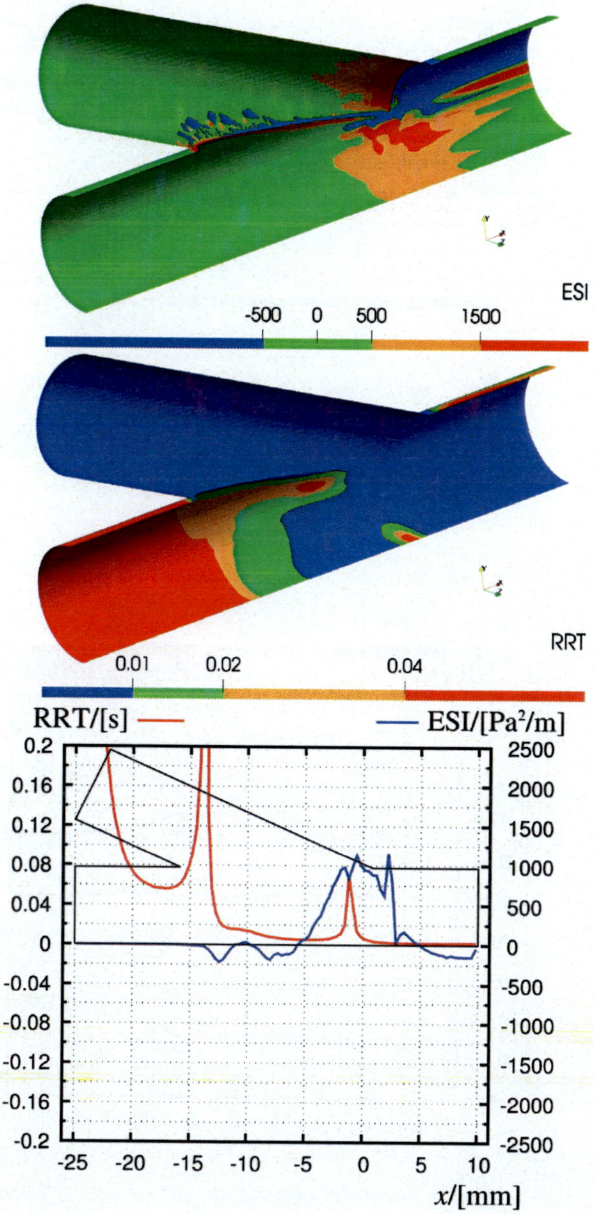

Fig. 4. Results for case (B): end-to-side distal anastomosis with the arterial blood flow in caudal direction only.

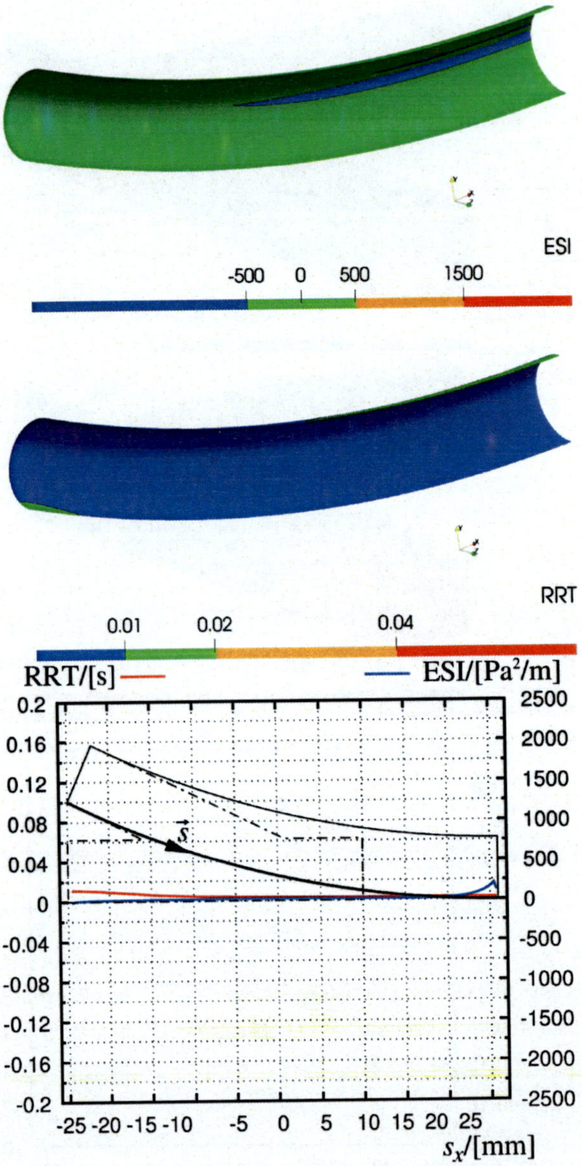

Fig. 5. Results for case (C): end-to-end distal anastomosis.

values of RRT in the range of 0.02 to 0.04s as high (orange zones in Figs. 3, 4 and 5) and above 0.04 s as extremely high (red zones in Figs. 3, 4 and 5).

In Case (A) (Fig. 3), when 20% of the total flowrate was directed cranially, it is visible that ESI (panel A) reached high values at all distal anastomosis sites where significant

IH was typically observed *in vivo* (suture line and artery floor). Also, high ESI values appear in the artery behind the anastomosis toe, while in all other regions ESI shows acceptable values. The RRT distribution (Panel B in Fig. 3) predicts IH in the arterial floor (in the region of moving stagnation point) and in the graft area near the anastomosis toe. High RRT values in the part of artery towards blockage are a consequence of small WSS due to a small flowrate in a large diameter artery. Finally, it follows from Panel C in Fig. 3 that both hypotheses predict IH in the artery floor since the regions of high ESI and high RRT overlap.

In Case (B) with only distal flow, the zone of high ESI becomes smaller in the vicinity of the anastomosis heel and larger near the toe. On the artery floor the zone of high ESI has moved caudally and the values of ESI and RRT are smaller than in Case (A). In the region of artery from blockage to the anastomosis, where there is practically no flow and WSS tends to zero, the RRT is high, indicating the thrombus formation. Obviously, in those cases it would be better to create an end-to-end instead of an end-to-side anastomosis to obtain a configuration without high ESI and RRT zones, as shown in Fig. 5.

IH in the region of the suture line is usually attributed to the surgical trauma, graft and artery compliance mismatch and elevated intramural stresses, but the results obtained in this study indicate that ESI should be considered as well.

A crucial question is how to prevent anastomotic site intimal hyperplasia? For this purpose, different strategies (mechanical, pharmacological, and gene therapies) against intimal hyperplasia have been suggested [2]. Several mechanical strategies based on the idea of changing the flow field to minimize low WSS regions by using different patches [15] showed a very limited or no success [14, 15]. An idea of a bifurcated graft [16] could solve the problem with artery floor IH, but it is likely unfeasible, due to the restrained space for graft placement which would lead to its unpredictable deformation in the lower extremity. Obtained results show that, at the artery floor, the zone of both high RRT around the moving stagnation point and high ESI (due to high WSSg) overlap. Such a condition is characteristic of the impinging jet flow [17], and it is present in all end-to-side anastomoses whenever the graft flow comes into the artery at a certain angle.

Considering this, one solution could be to replace a short segment of the artery at the distal anastomosis site with prosthesis, such that the T-shaped prefabricated graft bridges the resected part of the artery, as shown in Fig. 6.

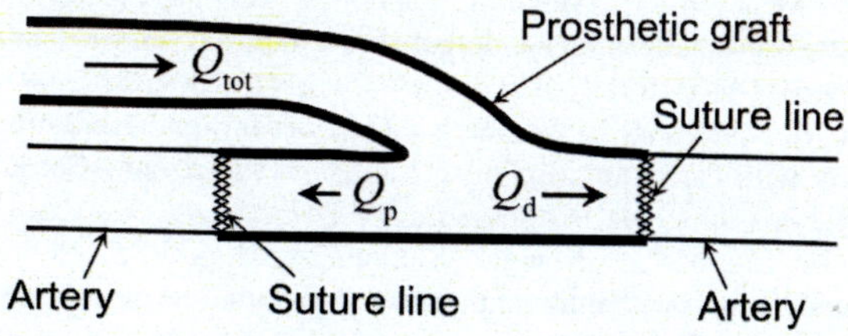

Fig. 6. Sketch of the prosthetic graft.

5 Limitations

Although we have used an idealized anastomosis model (suture line is a sharp edge, constant diameter of the artery, rigid wall, Newtonian model of blood), the usage a more realistic model would likely not change the global flow profile (impinging jet to the artery floor), but local changes near suture line could be expected.

6 Conclusion

The two indices, ESI and RRT, related to two hypotheses about the IH formation were calculated from the CFD solution of blood flow in the distal end-to-side and end-to-end anastomoses. Regions with high values of the newly proposed ESI in end-to-side anastomosis correlate very well with regions with significant IH observed in vivo. Interestingly, ESI shows high values in the vicinity of the suture line, offering an additional explanation for the IH initiation in that region. Based on the obtained results, a new solution for preventing end-to-side distal anastomosis stenosis was proposed. The solution includes the usage of prefabricated prosthetic graft, which would replace a part of the artery at the distal anastomotic site which is subjected to high ESI. The proposal requires further research.

References

1. Abularrage, C.J., Neville, R.F.: Infrainguinal revascularization. In: Surgical Pitfalls. Elsevier Inc., pp. 613–30 (2009). https://doi.org/10.1016/B978-141602951-9.50076-1
2. Collins, M.J., et al.: Therapeutic strategies to combat neointimal hyperplasia in vascular grafts. Expert Rev. Cardiovasc Ther. **10**(5), 635–647 (2012). https://doi.org/10.1586/erc.12.33
3. O'Brien, T.P., Grace, P., Walsh, M., Burke, P., McGloughlin, T.: Computational investigations of a new prosthetic femoral-popliteal bypass graft design. J. Vasc Surg. **42**(6), 1169–1175 (2005). https://doi.org/10.1016/j.jvs.2005.08.016
4. Keynton, R.S., Evancho, M.M., Sims, R.L., Rodway, N.V., Gobin, A., Rittgers, S.E.: Intimal hyperplasia and wall shear in arterial bypass graft distal anastomoses: an in vivo model study. J. Biomech. Eng. **123**(5), 464–473 (2001). https://doi.org/10.1115/1.1389461
5. Haruguchi, H., Teraoka, S.: Intimal hyperplasia and hemodynamic factors in arterial bypass and arteriovenous grafts: a review. J Artif Organs. **6**(4), 227–235 (2003). https://doi.org/10.1007/s10047-003-0232-x
6. Dolan, J.M., Meng, H., Singh, S., Paluch, R., Kolega, J.: High fluid shear stress and spatial shear stress gradients affect endothelial proliferation, survival, and alignment. Ann. Biomed. Eng. **39**(6), 1620–1631 (2011). https://doi.org/10.1007/s10439-011-0267-8
7. Peiffer, V., Sherwin, S.J., Weinberg, P.D.: Does low and oscillatory wall shear stress correlate spatially with early atherosclerosis? a systematic review. Cardiovasc Res. **99**(2), 242–250 (2013). https://doi.org/10.1093/cvr/cvt044
8. Meng, H., Tutino, V.M., Xiang, J., Siddiqui, A.: High WSS or low WSS? complex interactions of hemodynamics with intracranial aneurysm initiation, growth, and rupture: toward a unifying hypothesis. AJNR Am. J. Neuroradiol. **35**(7), 1254–1262 (2014). https://doi.org/10.3174/ajnr.A3558
9. Tuković, Ž., Karač, A., Cardiff, P., Jasak, H., iIvanković, A.: OpenFOAM finite volume solver for fluid-solid interaction. Trans. FAMENA **42**(3), 1–31 (2018). https://doi.org/10.21278/TOF.42301

10. Westerhof, N., Elzinga, G., Sipkema, P.: An artificial arterial system for pumping hearts. J. Appl. Physiol. **31**(5), 776–781 (1971). https://doi.org/10.1152/jappl.1971.31.5.776
11. Ku, D.N., Giddens, D.P., Phillips, D.J., Strandness, D.E., Jr.: Hemodynamics of the normal human carotid bifurcation: in vitro and in vivo studies. Ultrasound Med. Biol. **11**(1), 13–26 (1985). https://doi.org/10.1016/0301-5629(85)90003-1
12. Himburg, H.A., Grzybowski, D.M., Hazel, A.L., LaMack, J.A., Li, X.M., Friedman, M.H.: Spatial comparison between wall shear stress measures and porcine arterial endothelial permeability. Am J. Physiol. Heart Circ. Physiol. **286**(5), H1916–H1922 (2004). https://doi.org/10.1152/ajpheart.00897.2003
13. Donadoni, F., Pichardo-Almarza, C., Homer-Vanniasinkam, S., Dardik, A., Díaz-Zuccarini, V.: Multiscale, patient-specific computational fluid dynamics models predict formation of neointimal hyperplasia in saphenous vein grafts. J. Vasc Surg Cases Innov Tech. **6**(2), 292–306 (2020). https://doi.org/10.1016/j.jvscit.2019.09.009
14. Lemson, M.S., Tordoir, J.H., Daemen, M.J., Kitslaar, P.J.: Intimal hyperplasia in vascular grafts. Eur J. VascEndovasc Surg. **19**(4), 336–350 (2000). https://doi.org/10.1053/ejvs.1999.1040
15. Trubel, W., Schima, H., Czerny, M., Perktold, K., Schimek, M.G., Polterauer, P.: Experimental comparison of four methods of end-to-side anastomosis with expanded polytetrafluoroethylene. Br J Surg. **91**(2), 159–167 (2004). https://doi.org/10.1002/bjs.4388
16. Francis, L., Fischer, P.F., Bassiouny, H.S.: Annual Review of Fluid Mechanics **40**(1), 367-93 (2008)
17. Bassiouny, H.S., White, S., Glagov, S., Choi, E., Giddens, D.P., Zarins, C.K.: Anastomotic intimal hyperplasia: mechanical injury or flow induced. J. Vasc Surg. **15**(4), 708–16 (1992); discussion 716–7. https://doi.org/10.1067/mva.1992.33849

Non-invasive Functional Electrical Stimulation in Rehabilitation Engineering

Lana Popović-Maneski(✉)

Institute of Technical Sciences of SASA, Knez Mihailova 35/IV, Belgrade, Serbia
lana.popovic.maneski@itn.sanu.ac.rs

Abstract. Transcutaneous (non-invasive) functional electrical stimulation (FES) activates the ascending and descending neural pathways in persons with diminished sensory and motor control after a central nervous system (CNS) disease or injury. Application of FES in early phases of rehabilitation (acute and subacute) has a carry-over effect in decreasing motor impairment. FES is applied to the peripheral nervous system to activate the nerves and muscles, generate functional movements, and activate efferent and afferent neural pathways to close the biological motor-sensory loop. This promotes brain plasticity, the most important mechanism in rehabilitation after brain injuries. In the case of Spinal Cord Injuries (SCI), the functional recovery is less pronounced; however, the influence on the reduction of secondary complications of paralysis (e.g., loss of muscle bulk and strength, pressure sores, cardio-vascular deterioration, diminished gastric and urinary functioning, spasticity, reduced range of movement in joints, etc.) is pronounced. The most common applications of non-invasive FES are the restoration of standing and walking, the generation of cyclic movements for pedaling or rowing, and manipulation and grasping.

Keywords: Functional Electrical Stimulation · Rehabilitation · Neuroprosthesis

1 FES Fundamentals

Functional electrical stimulation is a method of external activation of sensory-motor systems to generate the missing or augment the diminished sensory or motor functions [1]. FES device can be described as a pacemaker that generates activities of the muscles in a time order that maximally mimics the activities of a healthy person when performing the same functions. The non-invasive FES pacemaker generates pulses of electrical charge that are delivered to the body via the electrodes on the skin. Electrical pulses generate action potentials (AP) in the motor and sensory nerve cells beneath the skin. The muscle receives both a direct descending AP and a reflexive AP initiated by the ascending AP in the spinal circuitry. The most efficient place to position the electrodes on the skin is close to the motor point, where the nerve endings enter the muscle and the descending path of AP is the shortest. If the muscle is denervated it can still be activated by surface FES, but with up to 3 orders of magnitude more power [2].

P. Bonačić Bartolin et al. (Eds.): BioMedVetMech 2022, IFMBE Proceedings 90, pp. 46–52, 2024.
https://doi.org/10.1007/978-3-031-42243-0_4

2 Beginnings of Non-invasive FES Neuroprostheses

The concept of neuroprosthesis (NP) based on FES was introduced by James Reswick and colleagues in the sixties of the last century [3]. The first non-invasive FES NP device was used to correct the drop foot syndrome in stroke patients in 1967 [4]. The device used two surface electrodes to stimulate the peroneal nerve and activate dorsiflexion based on the command signal from the switch placed under the heel (Fig. 1). The stimulation started when the switch detected the heel-off phase and lasted for the predefined time.

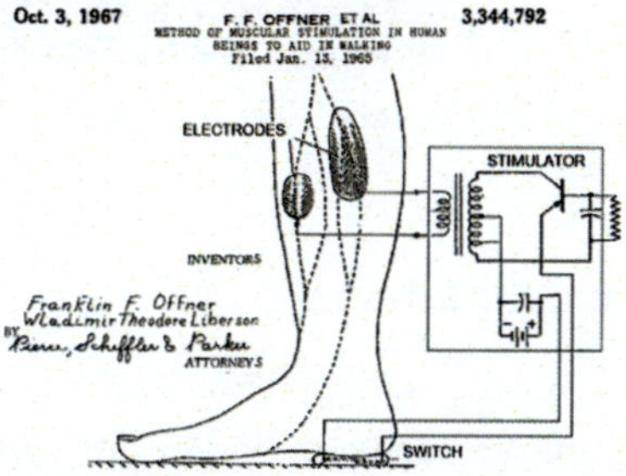

Fig. 1. First FES neuroprosthesis. Correction of the drop-foot syndrome. Modified from patent application US3344792A.

Between the sixties and eighties of the 20th century, the group from Ljubljana Faculty of Electrical Engineering, Slovenia, studied the application of multi-channel FES to help patients with leg paralysis to stand up and ambulate [5–7]. They stimulated major muscle groups (predominantly Quadriceps m., Hamstrings m., and Tibialis Anterior m.) with 6-channel programmable stimulators controlled by the hand switches. The patients learned how to timely control the stimulation and increase the efficiency by the proper posture of the upper body, which included hip hyperextension in the stance phases that led to biomechanical knee locking. They studied the use of this simple system in hundreds of subjects (spinal cord injury, cerebral palsy, stroke, etc.). In the nineties, the group from the University of Alberta, Edmonton, AB, Canada, and Miami Project to Cure Paralysis, USA, developed an automatic gait control for paraplegics by closed-loop control of 6 FES channels based on sensors for hip and knee angles (goniometers) and FSRs (force-resisting sensors) inside the shoes [8]. Paralyzed patients walked at speeds up to 1m/s, which is close to normal speeds, but the lack of proprioception was perceived as uncomfortable for the users (Fig. 2).

The first upper extremities NP allowed prehension and release for a person with tetraplegia and had a splint with a spring to close the hand and electrical stimulation of the thumb extensor to release the object [9].

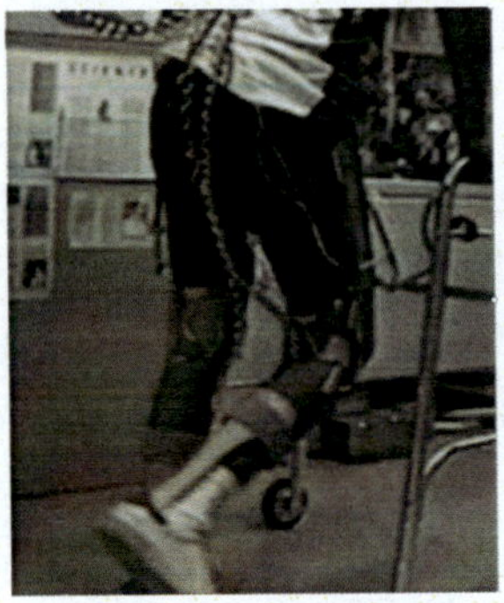

Fig. 2. Paraplegic patient walking with automatic FES gait based on closed-loop control with joints angle and GRF sensors

3 FES Neurorehabilitation

The use of peripheral FES as orthotic devices is still very limited due to several bottlenecks which prevent the popularization of this approach compared to implantable devices, such as time-consuming positioning of the electrodes and setting of parameters, fast muscle fatigue, etc. However, the peripheral FES became a standard tool for neurorehabilitation, especially when combined with intensive exercise and/or robotic aid.

FES is a powerful tool to enhance brain plasticity in the early phases of recovery (acute and sub-acute) after a brain injury, such as a stroke. FES is applied to the peripheral nervous system to activate the nerves and muscles, generate functional movements, and activate efferent and afferent neural pathways to close the biological motor-sensory loop (Fig. 3) even when the motor command is missing or compromised. The brain can change, adapt and regain the lost functions with intensive exercise. Popovic et al. [10] showed that a 3-week FES program for grasping in the acute phase after stroke significantly increases functions, with a carry-over effect after 12 months. Application of FES in chronic patients after 12 months leads to non-significant improvements.

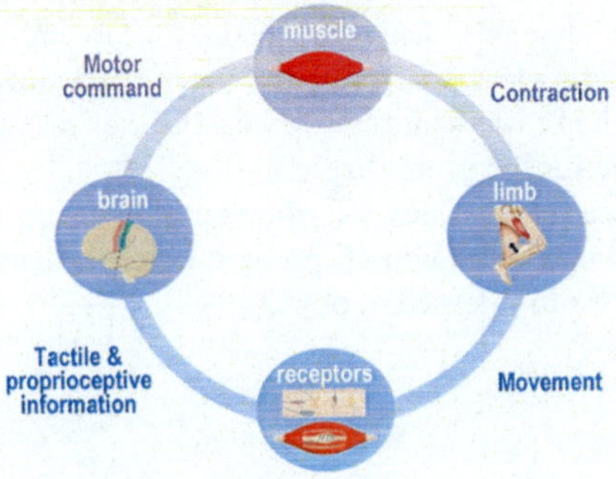

Fig. 3. Biological motor-sensory loop

In the case of Spinal Cord Injuries (SCI), less significant functional recovery can be achieved at spinal levels close to the level of injury; however, the influence on the reduction of secondary complications of paralysis (e.g., loss of muscle bulk and strength, pressure sores, cardio-vascular deterioration, diminished gastric and urinary functioning, spasticity, reduced range of movement in joints, etc.) is well pronounced. Table 1 summarizes the benefits of FES in stroke and SCI patients and the general constraints of the technology.

Table 1. Peripheral FES benefits and constraints

	Benefits	Constraints
SPINAL CORD INJURIES ---STROKE----	Physical activity, endurance, muscle power	Fast muscle fatigue
	The practice of a range of motion	Time-consuming positioning of electrodes
	Improved cardiovascular health	The time-consuming setting of parameters
	Enhance of brain plasticity	Personalization of stimulation sequence
	Reduction of spasticity	Only superficial muscles can be activated
	Prevention of pressure sores	
	Prevention of osteoporosis	
	Reduction of urinary infections	

Currently available commercial devices are general-purpose stimulators with programmable stimulation sequences and cables for connection to multi-use electrodes [11–15] or compact systems focused on the correction of the drop-foot [16–18] or grasp [19–21]. In addition, sometimes FES is combined with robotic systems to provide guided cyclic or target-oriented movements and assist high-intensity and repetitive exercise of coordinated limb motion. Examples are FES-cycling [22–26] and FES-rowing [25] ergometers, FES-walking, or grasping combined with lower and upper extremity exoskeletons [27].

4 FES Constraints and Solutions

Although FES can bring many benefits to the user, the complexity of use for this technology is still not at the level that allows acceptable setup time for the rehabilitation of many different patients in clinical settings or prolonged periods of use as an orthotic device. Reduction of setup time can be achieved with garments with incorporated electrodes, preferably dry electrodes that do not require a layer of sticky gel in contact with skin, as shown in Fig. 4E. However, this is feasible only in lower extremities, where the muscles are big and small mistakes in electrode positioning do not lead to a drastic reduction of selectivity. In the upper extremities, muscles are narrow and very close, where differences of less than 1 cm for electrode positioning make a noticeable difference in the resulting movement. In this case, a promising solution is the use of muti-pad electrodes [21, 28, 29], as shown in Fig. 4C. Multi-pad electrodes allow the selection of one or more

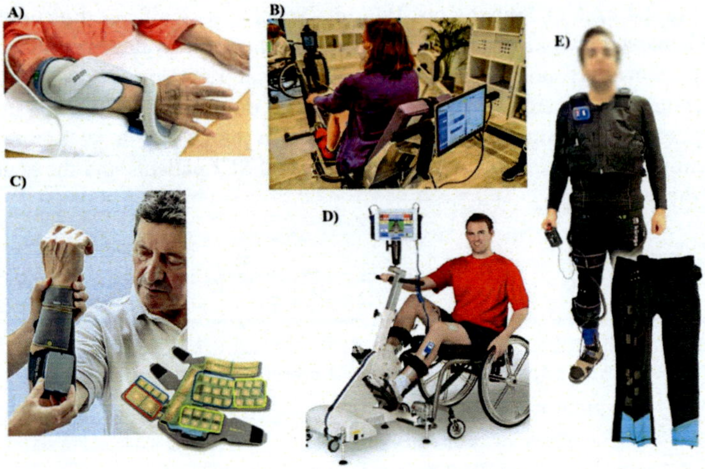

Fig. 4. FES devices: A) NESS H200, Bioness, USA B) Concept 2 rower with Motimove stimulator by Kurage, France, C) Feasia Grasp, Fesia Technology, Spain, D) RT300, Restorative Therapies, USA, E) Neuroskin, Kurage, France.

distinct active pads to produce the desired movement. On the other hand, applications on the upper extremities do not deal with a problem of fast muscle fatigue, as high-intensity stimulations of lower extremity muscles. Muscle fatigue is very fast due to FES because of the high rates of motor unit recruitments, all units being recruited simultaneously, and a reversed recruitment order compared to CNS strategies. Surface-distributed asynchronous stimulation [30–32] is one way to delay muscle fatigue, later named spatially distributed sequential stimulation (SDSS). This method uses four closely positioned smaller electrodes instead of one large electrode to deliver stimulation pulses at four times lower frequencies each, resulting in the same level of fused contraction and up to 250% longer fatigue periods. The rationale behind this approach is that each small electrode activates a different pool of motor units of the same muscle or the synergistic muscles and this way mimics the natural strategy of the CNS.

5 Conclusion

FES is a powerful tool for rehabilitation after a disease or injury of the central nervous system. The most significant effects are achieved in the acute phases. However, the devices based on FES are still not in the development stage where this technology can be introduced in everyday practice in typical clinical environments because of the constraints of time-consuming setup, fast muscle fatigue, and, sometimes, inconvenient generated sensations. Therefore, special care has to be taken to ensure that the devices based on FES are easy to use, fast to set up, and allow a certain level of autonomy in adjusting and personalizing the parameters to each user.

References

1. Popović, D.B., Popović-Maneski, L.: Neuroprosthesis and functional electrical stimulation (Peripheral). Handbook of Neuroengineering. Springer Singapore, Singapore, pp. 1–40 (2022). https://doi.org/10.1007/978-981-15-2848-4_51-1
2. Mayr, W., et al.: Functional Electrical Stimulation (FES) of denervated muscles: existing and prospective technological solutions. Basic Appl. Myol. **12**(6), 287–290 (2002)
3. Reswick, J.B., Ko, W., Vodovnik, L., Mc Leod, W., Crochetiere, W.: On the cybernetic restoration of human function in paralysis. In: Advances in External Control of Human Extremities II, pp. 3–13, Published by ETAN, Belgrade, Yugoslavia (1967). Popović, D.B. (Ed.) "Advances in External Control of Human Extremities I-X", CD, Aalborg University, 2002. ISBN 8790562089, 9788790562083
4. Liberson, W.T.: Functional electrotherapy: stimulation of the peroneal nerve synchronized with the swing phase of the gait of hemiplegic patients. Arch Phys. Med. **42**, 101–105 (1961)
5. Bajd, T., Kralj, A., Turk, R., Benko, H., Šega, J.: Use of functional electrical stimulation in the rehabilitation of patients with incomplete spinal cord injuries. J. Biomed. Eng. **11**(2), 96–102 (1989)
6. Kralj, A., Vodovnik, L.: Functional electrical stimulation of the extremities: part 1. J. Med. Eng. Technol. **1**(1), 12–15 (1977)
7. Strojnik, P., Kralj, A., Uršič, I.: Programmed six-channel electrical stimulator for complex stimulation of leg muscles during walking. IEEE Trans. Biomed. Eng. **2**, 112–116 (1979)
8. Kostov, A., et al.: Machine learning in control of functional electrical stimulation systems for locomotion. IEEE Transactions on Biomedical Engineering **42**(6), 541–551 (1995)
9. Long, C., Masciarelli, V.D.: An electrophysiologic splint for the hand. Arch. Phys. Med. RehabiL. **44**, 499503 (1963)
10. Popovic, D.B., et al.: Therapy of paretic arm in hemiplegic subjects augmented with a neural prosthesis: a cross-over study. Canadian J. Physiology and Pharmacology **82**(8–9), 749–756 (2004)
11. Valtin, M., Kociemba, K., Behling, C., Kuberski, B., Becker, S., Schauer, T.: RehaMovePro: A versatile mobile stimulation system for transcutaneous FES applications. European J. Translational Myology **26**(3), (2016)
12. Negard, N.O., Schauer, T., de Gersigny, J., Hesse, S., Raisch, J.: Application programming interface and PC control for the 8 channel stimulator MOTIONSTIM8. In: 10th Annual Conference of the International Functional Electrical Stimulation Society: IFESS 2005, pp. 27–29 (2005)
13. Popović-Maneski, L., Mateo, S.: MotiMove: multi-purpose transcutaneous functional electrical stimulator. Artif. Organs **46**(10), 1970–1979 (2022)
14. https://stiwell.medel.com/stiwell-products/stiwell-med4/application-areas/fes-after-a-stroke. Accessed 1 Oct. 2022
15. https://www.myndtec.com/clinicians/myndmove-therapy/. Accessed 1 Oct. 2022
16. https://www.l300go.com/. Accessed 1 Oct. 2023
17. https://www.myndtec.com/product/myndstep-stimulator/. Accessed 1 Oct. 2023
18. Malešević, J., et al.: A decision support system for electrode shaping in multi-pad FES foot drop correction. J. Neuroengineering and Rehabilitation **14**(1), 1–14 (2017)
19. https://media.ottobock.com/_web-site/orthotics/bioness-h200-wireless-system/646d1290_en_master-01-1803w_.int.pdf. Accessed 1 Oct. 2023
20. Paolo, M., et al.: Hand Glove FES Device (Re-Grasp) in Neurological Patients Affected by Upper Limb Disability. Int. J. Neurorehabilitation **6**, 358 (2019)
21. https://fesiatechnology.com/en/. Accessed 1 Oct. 2023
22. https://www.musclepower.com/pdf/ERGYS3OperatorManual.pdf. Accessed 1 Oct. 2023

23. https://restorative-therapies.com/ifes-systems/rt300/. Accessed 1 Oct. 2023
24. https://myolyn.com/for-home/overview/. Accessed 1 Oct. 2023
25. https://kurage.fr/en/return-to-effort-kurage-rehabilitation/. Accessed 1 Oct. 2023
26. https://berkelbike.com/product/fes-functional-electrical-stimulation/. Accessed 1 Oct. 2023
27. Anaya, F., Thangavel, P., Yu, H.: Hybrid FES–robotic gait rehabilitation technologies: a review on mechanical design, actuation, and control strategies. Int. J. Intell. Robotics Appl. **2**(1), 1–28 (2018)
28. Malešević, N.M., et al.: A multi-pad electrode based functional electrical stimulation system for restoration of grasp. J. Neuroengineering Rehabilitation **9**(1), 66 (2012)
29. Popović-Maneski, L., et al.: Multi-pad electrode for effective grasping: design. IEEE Trans. Neural Syst. Rehabil. Eng. **21**(4), 648–654 (2013)
30. Popović, L., Malešević, N.: Muscle fatigue of quadriceps in paraplegics: comparison between single vs. multi-pad electrode surface stimulation. In: Proc of IEEE EMBC, Minneapolis, MN, Sept 2–6, pp. 6785–6788 (2009)
31. Malešević, N.M., Popović, L.Z., Schwirtlich, L., Popović, D.B.: Distributed low-frequency functional electrical stimulation delays muscle fatigue compared to conventional stimulation. Muscle Nerve **42**(4), 556–562 (2010)
32. Popović Maneski, L., Malešević, N.M., Savić, A.M., Keller, T., Popović, D.B.: Surface-distributed low-frequency asynchronous stimulation delays fatigue of stimulated muscles. Muscle & Nerve **48**(6), 930–937 (2013)

Low-Back Pain Patients Classification Based on sEMG Activation Patterns Detection

Vedran Srhoj-Egekher[1](✉), Mario Cifrek[1], and Stanislav Peharec[2]

[1] Faculty of Electrical Engineering and Computing, University of Zagreb, Zagreb, Croatia
vedran.srhoj-egekher@fer.hr

[2] Faculty of Medicine, University of Rijeka, Rijeka, Croatia

Abstract. Low back pain (LBP) diagnostic challenge to assigning patients into more specific groups has been detected as one of the key obstacles in ensuring successful rehabilitation treatments. Novel approaches treat LBP patients as a non-homogeneous group where a more individualized approach is proposed, thus leading to a need for an effective subgrouping. In this paper, the possibility to differentiate chronic low back patients (CLBP) from LBP patients with radiculopathy (RLBP), by means of surface electromyography (sEMG), was examined. A feature model based on muscle activation patterns was proposed by measuring time distances between consecutive pairs of distinguished myoelectric events. For each sEMG channel, median and 90th percentile values of time distances were calculated. This procedure was applied to six simple raw features: zero crossing (ZC), signal slope change (SSC), Willison amplitude (WAMP), variance (VAR), relative variance difference (RVD), and permutation entropy (PE). The classification differentiation task (CLBP vs. RLBP) was accomplished by employing support vector machines (SVM) and nearest neighbor (kNN) classifier variants. The presented approach demonstrated consistent high-accuracy classification results (0.90) for the given CLBP and RLBP subgrouping. The obtained results suggest that muscle activation patterns are worth further exploring as part of interpretable LBP patients' subgrouping efforts.

Keywords: Low-back pain · Classification · Activation patterns · Subgrouping

1 Introduction

Low back pain (LBP) is a global health problem with a significant socio-economic impact. One of the key challenges in medical diagnostics and treatments is formulated with a real-life fact that about 90% of patients, with LBP, are being no better diagnosed and categorized, but by stating that their LBP issues are *non-specific*. This poses significant limitations in ensuring proper rehabilitation procedures. Consequently, this led to hypothesizing that (non-specific) LBP patients are not a homogeneous group, but a more individualized approach is needed to account for the diversity and complexity behind them [1]. Furthermore, among patients with LBP disorders, 5–10% of patients can usually be related to radicular syndrome [2].

P. Bonačić Bartolin et al. (Eds.): BioMedVetMech 2022, IFMBE Proceedings 90, pp. 53–59, 2024.
https://doi.org/10.1007/978-3-031-42243-0_5

In this paper, we examine the possibilities of subgrouping LBP patients by analyzing different muscle activation and trigger events. It is observed in other studies that patients with LBP tend to exhibit altered or irregular muscle activation patterns compared to healthy subjects [3, 4]. However, there is still no unambiguous proof of whether such irregular patterns can directly support differentiation within the LBP group itself.

2 Materials and Methods

2.1 Subjects

Three different groups of male volunteers were involved in this research concerning the presence of low back pain: healthy subjects (HS), patients with chronic low back pain (CLBP), and low back pain patients with radiculopathy (RLBP). Inclusion criteria for CLBP were defined as daily or almost daily pain that lasted at least three months before measurements [5]. For RLBP patients, the main inclusion criteria were clinical symptoms of radiculopathy with a positive Lasegue sign on one side lasting at least fourteen days [6]. Ninety-one subjects were divided with a share of 40.7%, 31.9%, and 27.4% among HS, CLBP, and RLBP groups, respectively. Demographic and biometric statistics did not show any significant differences among groups with respect to age, height, weight, and BMI.

2.2 Measurement Protocol and Data Acquisition

The isometric trunk extension exercise, in the configuration of the Roman chair (a variant of the Biering-Sørensen test [7]), was selected as a muscle activation procedure for the onset of muscle fatigue (see Fig. 1). FREEEMG (BTS, Milano, Italy) wireless surface EMG system was utilized for myoelectric muscle activity recording.

Four sEMG channels were placed in the paraspinal lumbar region over the upper lumbar erector spinae (ULES) and lower lumbar erector spinae (LLES) muscle sites, bilaterally (left and right) with respect to the vertical spine axis (see Fig. 1). The subject's upper body weight was used to induce muscle fatigue. The subject was asked to sustain the isometric contraction as long as possible or until a maximum exercise duration of 180 s was reached.

2.3 Feature Extraction

A set of six simple raw features was chosen to capture LBP-related myoelectric activation patterns, namely: zero crossing (ZC), signal slope change (SSC), Willison amplitude (WAMP), variance (VAR), relative variance difference (RVD), and permutation entropy (PE). Based on the extended analysis presented in [8], the respective set of features was detected and confirmed as the best one for the sEMG-based analysis of LBP characteristics. All features were calculated in the time domain (TD). However, features tend to carry different types of information: frequency-related (ZC, SSC, WAMP), energy-related (VAR, RVD), or non-linear (PE). Such composition of feature characteristics enables tackling different aspects of LBP expressions via sEMG.

Considering the sEMG signals' non-stationary and non-linear properties [9], smaller time chunks of sEMG signals were consecutively analyzed, as presented in [8].

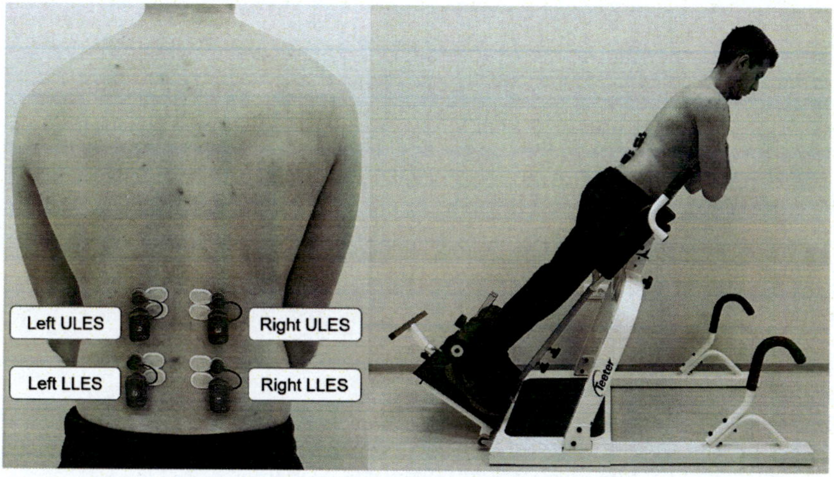

Fig. 1. The position of sEMG electrodes in the lumbar region (left). Tilting device in the Roman chair configuration used for trunk extension exercise (right).

3 Feature Modeling

3.1 Reference Models

First, a baseline model for comparative classification analysis was chosen based on the comprehensive feature modeling, supporting the interpretability of classification results, as presented in [8]. The proposed concept consists of several LBP contextual feature groups: coordination measures, namely, co-activation triggers, trends, and fatigue-related indices.

3.2 Inter-event Time Distance Measure

Following the simple concept of detecting co-activation triggers, as described in [8], a new metric, based on these trigger events, was introduced and presented in this paper. Namely, a time distance between each of two consecutive trigger events is calculated, for each sEMG channel separately (see Fig. 2). The procedure for calculating the respective inter-event time distance measure is defined with the following steps:

1. Find the prominent localized peaks (higher than 90-percentile peak height and with a minimum distance of 250 ms between two consecutive peaks), for a selected raw feature (ZC, SSC, WAMP, VAR, RVD, PE), for each channel ch_i with $i = 1$ to 4.
2. Select one channel and iterate across all maxima (peaks) for that channel and calculate the time distance between each pair of two consecutive peaks.
3. For each array of such calculated inter-event time distances, calculate the median and 90th percentile time-distance value, per channel separately.
4. Repeat the procedure for all channels.
5. Repeat the procedure for all raw features.

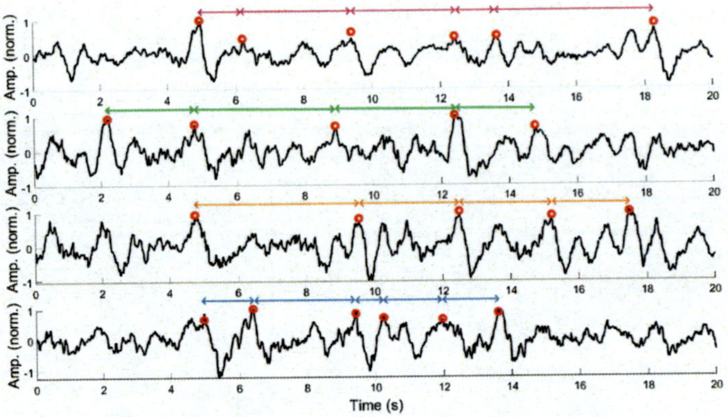

Fig. 2. Inter-event time distance examples, for several selected consecutive trigger events, for one CLBP patient, based on the RVD feature. All four channels left ULES, left LLES, right ULES, and right LLES, from top to bottom, respectively, are shown.

3.3 Feature Selection and Classification Models

The feature selection procedure was based on the neighborhood component analysis (NCA) technique [10]. Two clear benefits were gained with this approach: features remain in the original domain (thus supporting easier resulting models' interpretation) and a significant reduction in the number of feature model components.

Four different classifiers and respective variants were employed in this paper (see Table 1 and Table 2). Support vector machines (SVM) with its two variants, quadratic and cubic SVM with soft-margin separation criterion, then, k-nearest neighbor (kNN) classifier with its fine resolution ($k = 1$) variant, and ensemble subspace method based on medium resolution ($k = 10$) kNN classifier, were selected. The respective classifiers had demonstrated to be the optimal choice among a wider range of different classifiers and their variants (twenty-three classification models examined) for different binary (two-class) LBP differentiation tasks (HS vs. LBP, HS vs. RLBP, HS vs. CLBP, and CLBP vs. RLBP), as presented in [8].

Classification tasks and model verification were performed on a full data set in a ten-fold cross-validation manner.

As presented in Table 1 and Table 2, the extended reference models (III) and (VII) incorporated new inter-event distance measure features into the existing co-activation triggers reference models (II) and (VI), respectively. For models (IV) and (VII), only new inter-event time distance measures (median and 90th percentile) as features were employed.

Table 1. Two-class classification (HS vs. LBP) accuracy results (with ten-fold cross-validation) for different feature models are shown. The reference model (I), consisting of all feature groups (All), and model (II) consisting only of co-activation triggers (CA), are shown. New classification results for the extended model (III), including new inter-even time distance values and a new inter-event distance model only (IV), are shown next.

Classifier	(I) Ref. Model (All)	(II) Ref. Model (CA)	(III) Extended ref. Model (CA)	(IV) Inter-event distance model
Quadratic SVM	**0.93**	0.80	0.80	0.76
Cubic SVM	**0.94**	0.87	0.80	0.79
Fine kNN	**0.89**	0.83	0.87	0.77
Subspace kNN	**0.91**	0.84	0.88	0.83
No. of NCA components	20	12	27	15

Table 2. Two-class classification (CLBP vs. RLBP) accuracy results (with ten-fold cross-validation) for different feature models are shown. The reference model (V), consisting of all feature groups (All), and model (VI) consisting only of co-activation triggers (CA), are shown. New classification results for the extended model (VII), including new inter-even time distance values and a new inter-event distance model only (VIII), are shown next.

Classifier	(V) Ref. Model (All)	(VI) Ref. Model (CA)	(VII) Extended ref. Model (CA)	(VIII) Inter-event distance model
Quadratic SVM	0.82	0.68	**0.88**	0.86
Cubic SVM	0.83	0.76	0.86	**0.90**
Fine kNN	0.89	0.66	0.88	**0.90**
Subspace kNN	0.87	0.69	0.81	**0.90**
No. of NCA components	14	9	9	10

4 Results

Two-class classification tasks for HS vs. LBP differentiation (see Table 1) demonstrated that the comprehensive reference model (I) outperformed the remaining models based on single feature groups constructed around co-activation triggers and new inter-event distance measures (II)–(III). The best accuracy results for (I) are >0.90 across most of the classifiers, whereas the best classification accuracy results for the remaining models are obtained for the extended model (III), with results of 0.80 for SVM classifiers and 0.87 and 0.88 for fine kNN and subspace kNN classifiers, respectively.

Classification results for CLBP vs. RLBP classification task (see Table 2) confirm the limited accuracy obtained with the reference model (V), ranging from 0.82–0.87, where the best classification result was obtained with the subspace kNN classifier, similarly as reported in [8]. Significantly deteriorated accuracy results were obtained for the reference model based only on the co-activation triggers feature group (VI), ranging from 0.66–0.76. Best-performing results were obtained with the newly proposed model based on the inter-event time distance model with classification accuracy results ranging from 0.86–0.90, where the following classifiers, cubic SVM, fine kNN, and subspace kNN resulted in an accuracy of 0.90.

5 Discussion

A subgrouping of LBP patients was presented as the major challenge in the analysis of LBP. To verify the proposed inter-event time distance model in tackling this challenge, a differentiation of two LBP groups at hand, CLBP and RLBP, was examined as deemed to be a relevant task for analyzing subgrouping potential.

In previous studies reported by other authors [3, 4] the possibility of analyzing muscle activation patterns in different domains (i.e., different feature vector spaces) was shown to provide additional insight into LBP characteristics expressed via sEMG. In our previous study [8], the focus was primarily on detecting the muscle activation synchronization patterns among different muscle sites (muscle locations), resulting in the concept of co-activation triggers scores. In this study, the focus was put on analyzing the muscle activation patterns within the muscle site itself (i.e., for each sEMG channel separately). The starting hypothesis was based on the evidence that different LBP-related conditions result in different muscle activation patterns. This can be connected to different neuromotor control coding strategies required to compensate for insufficiencies and to sustain muscle contraction [1].

Differentiation between the HS and LBP groups poses a certain complexity due to the LBP group not being homogeneous (it consists of CLBP and RLBP groups). This explains the necessity to engage more complex feature models to tackle samples' variations in this classification task, resulting in the respective results presented in Table 2. Thus, the best results demonstrated by the reference model (I) were expected, whereas the simplest feature groups, (II) and (IV), modeling just a single aspect of muscle activations related to LBP, resulted in the least accurate results.

On the other hand, CLBP and RLBP groups are more homogeneous, however, this requires more specific differentiators between the groups to be detected and employed for successful subgrouping. Following this reasoning, the comprehensive models presented with the reference model (V) failed in resulting consistently in high classification accuracy, with the best accuracy obtained of 0.89, whereas, relatively simple models, especially the newly proposed inter-event distance model (VIII) demonstrated consistently very good classification accuracy results of 0.90, across multiple employed classifiers. Co-activation triggers model (VI), as originally presented in [8], was not able to adequately perform the differentiation task for the CLBP vs. RLBP pair.

6 Conclusion

A new feature model for differentiation between CLBP and RLBP groups, based on measuring time distances between distinguished muscle activation events, was presented. A simple procedure based on an isometric trunk extension exercise and only four sEMG channels employed, resulted in 0.90 classification accuracy for the given task, consistently across several classifiers.

These promising results will drive future work with a focus on establishing deeper relations within muscle activation patterns and triggers' firing presence or absence, with the aim to incorporate these findings into the single comprehensive LBP features model, thus further supporting the construction of interpretable LBP models.

References

1. Hodges, P.W.: Pain and motor control: from the laboratory to rehabilitation. J. Electromyogr. Kinesiol. **21**(2), 220–228 (2011)
2. Bardin, L.D., King, P., Maher, C.G.: Diagnostic triage for low back pain: a practical approach for primary care. Med. J. Aust. **206**(6), 268–273 (2017)
3. Newcomer, K.L., Jacobson, T.D., Gabriel, D.A., Larson, D.R., Brey, R.H., An, K.N.: Muscle activation patterns in subjects with and without low back pain. Arch. Phys. Med. Rehabil. **83**(6), 816–821 (2002)
4. Hu, Y., Siu, S.H., Mak, J.N., Luk, K.D.: Lumbar muscle electromyographic dynamic topography during flexion-extension. J. Electromyogr. Kinesiol. **20**(2), 246–255 (2010)
5. van der Hulst, M., Vollenbroek-Hutten, M.M., Rietman, J.S., Hermens, H.J.: Lumbar and abdominal muscle activity during walking in subjects with chronic low back pain: support of the "guarding" hypothesis? J. Electromyogr. Kinesiol. **20**(1), 31–38 (2010)
6. Reger, S.I., et al.: Classification of large array surface myoelectric potentials from subjects with and without low back pain. J. Electromyogr. Kinesiol. **16**(4), 392–401 (2006)
7. Biering-Sørensen, F.I.N.: Physical measurements as risk indicators for low-back trouble over a one-year period. Spine **9**(2), 106–119 (1984)
8. Srhoj-Egekher, V., Cifrek, M., Peharec, S.: Feature modeling for interpretable low back pain classification based on surface EMG. IEEE Access **10**, 73702–73727 (2022)
9. Karlsson, S., Yu, J., Akay, M.: Time-frequency analysis of myoelectric signals during dynamic contractions: a comparative study. IEEE Trans. Biomed. Eng. **47**(2), 228–238 (2000)
10. Goldberger, J., Hinton, G.E., Roweis, S., Salakhutdinov, R.R.: Neighbourhood components analysis. In: Advances in Neural Information Processing Systems 17 (2004)

Check for updates

Wireless Device for Biomedical Signal Acquisition with Dry Electrodes on an e-Bike

L. Klaić(✉), I. Čuljak, A. Stanešić, I. Vrhoci, P. Šajinović, M. Cifrek, and H. Džapo

Faculty of Electrical Engineering and Computing, University of Zagreb, Zagreb, Croatia
{luka.klaic,ivana.culjak,antonio.stanesic,ivan.vrhoci, patrik.sajinovic,mario.cifrek,hrvoje.dzapo}@fer.hr

Abstract. With the advent of ubiquitous computing and the widespread availability of advanced low-power embedded processors and systems-on-chip (SoCs), wearable devices find their way into a large number of practical applications. Recent technological advances enabled the widespread use of various types of biomedical devices for monitoring everyday human activities. Fitness trackers are now particularly popular devices that provide users valuable and useful insights into their state of fitness, health, and wellness, thus enabling a better quality of life and serving an important public health goal of preventing unwanted health conditions later in life. On the other hand, there has been a rising interest in e-mobility and particularly micromobility, not only in the context of green transition and global climate changes, but also because of the rising awareness of the importance of physical activity in everyday life. This paper presents an innovative measurement solution that integrates a biomedical signal tracker into a modern design of an e-bike to allow automatic signal acquisition, without the need for a driver to wear any device directly on a body. The main challenge was how to design a system that would have a minimal impact on user experience and allow biosignals acquisition from bicycle handles. The proposed system consists of a specialized biomedical analog front-end, dry electrodes in direct contact with skin, a processor unit, and Bluetooth Low Energy interface to a smart device. It was experimentally demonstrated that the proposed device is capable of acquiring respiration signals, as well as electrocardiogram (ECG) signals during normal cycling operation with a minimum impact on user experience.

Keywords: biomedical instrumentation · biomedical signal acquisition · dry electrodes · wireless sensors · electric bicycles · Bluetooth Low Energy

1 Introduction

Recent advances in wearable sensing technologies, followed by constant miniaturization of hardware and sensor integration, allow their use in everyday applications, such as security, gaming, entertainment, defense, or the transport industry [1]. Furthermore, through low-power solutions and the use of surface electrodes, such sensor systems can be adapted for non-invasive health monitoring. From assisted living to sports gadgets, smart wearable devices make daily health tracking possible. Especially in the

P. Bonačić Bartolin et al. (Eds.): BioMedVetMech 2022, IFMBE Proceedings 90, pp. 60–72, 2024.
https://doi.org/10.1007/978-3-031-42243-0_6

past decade, alongside technological improvements, a significant upward trend in the wearable devices market is present (Fig. 1).

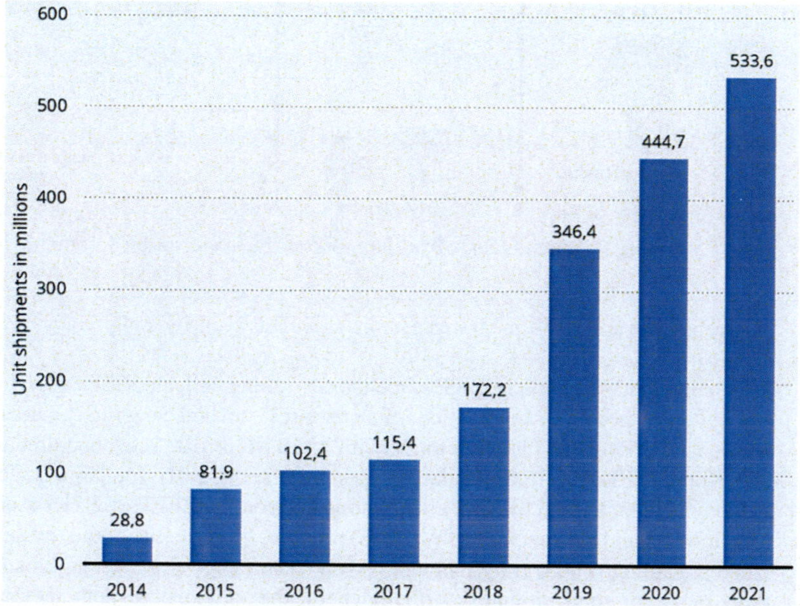

Fig. 1. Total wearable device unit shipments worldwide from 2014 to 2021 in millions, [2].

When considering monitoring their everyday living surroundings, it is important to allow subjects to move freely and independently of the sensor platform. Hence, communication with the monitoring system is nowadays preferably wireless in order to minimize the impact on normal user activities. Therefore, typical modern wearable biomedical systems consist of multiple nodes and are usually referred to as Wireless Body Area Networks (WBANs), meaning that all wireless devices are closely related to a human body as a hub where all measurement data are acquired and processed. An example of a modern WBAN architecture for biomedical monitoring is shown in Fig. 2. Such networks may include Intra-BAN communication between wireless sensors (level 1), when a special kind of intrabody communication (IBC) is used to enable more energy efficient and more secure intra-sensor communication [3]. On the next level, the special coordinator – master node, mediates Inter-BAN communication between the master node and personal devices. Beyond-BAN communication connects the local network to the Internet on the last level [4].

Communication between different nodes can be established by means of different technologies, each offering specific characteristics, advantages, and disadvantages. The most suitable one is chosen depending on the concrete application, when different technical requirements are evaluated and compared, such as the coverage area range, data transfer rate, power consumption, etc. In addition, some medical applications require

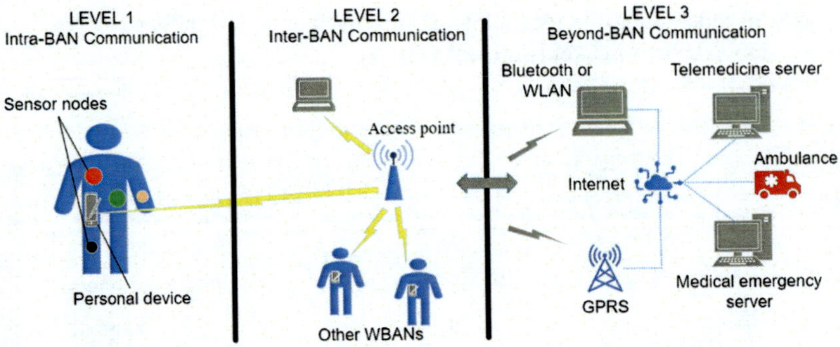

Fig. 2. Wireless Body Area Networks architecture, adapted from [4].

high reliability and real-time transmission, as well as security and privacy of transmitted data [4].

Thanks to its sleep mode, ZigBee technology, along with the IEEE 802.15.4 standard, is a suitable choice for applications that require a several years-long battery life and secure networking. On the other hand, with its 10 Mbps data rate compared to Zigbee's 250 Kbps, IEEE 802.15.6 standard is designed specifically for large-scale WBANs. Although characterized by high energy consumption, the IEEE 802.11 set of standards for wireless local area networks (WLANs) provides high-quality audio transmission and video streaming. The Ultra-wideband (UWB) technology provides high bandwidth for short-range communication [5]. Although being the only reliable method of localization, it is not the first choice when it comes to wearable applications. ANT protocol, Zarlink technology, and Rubee protocol are other examples of emerging standards for wellness and health monitoring [4].

Operating in the 2.4 GHz ISM (Industrial, Scientific and Medical) band, the consumer Bluetooth standard covers ranging from 1 to 30 m [6], with a maximum data rate of 3 Mbps, at the same time maintaining high levels of security without the need of a line-of-sight positioning of connected devices [4]. With 1 Mbps speed, its derived version, Bluetooth Low Energy (BLE), achieves half the power consumption whilst using low duty cycle operation [7]. Since it is particularly dedicated to wearable low-bandwidth applications and device configuration, it will be used to connect the central wireless biomedical system (WBS) to a personal computer or mobile phone.

The rest of the paper is organized as follows: Sect. 2. Surveys the developed system. Next, Sect. 3. Brings examples of the obtained results. Lastly, Sect. 4. Brings a conclusion.

2 System Overview

The goal of the system is to provide monitoring of cyclists' ECG and respiration by means of dry electrodes.

A set of requirements for the developed WBS node is shown in Fig. 3. The requirements encompass the following: (1) the interface for obtaining respiration rate from bioimpedance, as well as ECG signal, by means of dry electrodes designed following guidelines presented in [8], (2) the interface for obtaining current bicycle acceleration and orientation, (3) data acquisition (DAQ) hardware with analog preprocessing and analog-to-digital conversion, (4) digital processing on a microprocessor, (5) communication with external systems via different debug and production interfaces (wired and wireless) to the back-end platforms, such as a personal computer or a mobile phone. Moreover, (6) battery or wired power supply must be implemented, with low-power design in mind to maximize battery autonomy during long-term measurements.

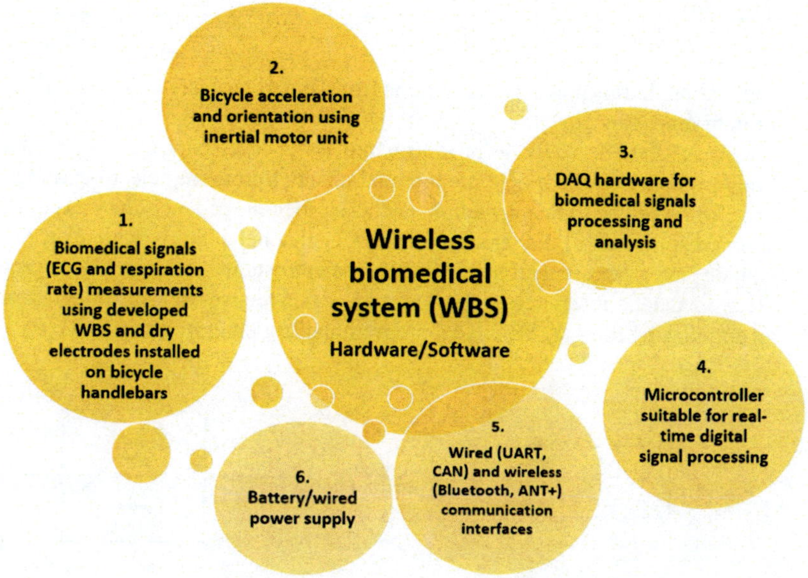

Fig. 3. Technical specification of a common specialized WBS node.

2.1 Analog Biomedical Front-End

To obtain all signals of interest from the subject, activity monitoring demands a combination of different sensors, combined to form a multimodal system. For a purpose of system development, few specialized integrated circuits were considered, tested, and compared (Maxim Integrated MAX3000x, MAX301xx, and MAX861xx). The goal was to evaluate SoC that can be used to measure bioimpedance, as well as biopotentials – ECG. In Table 1, an overview of the different capabilities of ultra-low power, single-channel integrated analog front-ends (AFEs) from the MAX3000x series is given.

Due to its multi-functionality, MAX30001 AFE is a solution for a wide range of medical applications, such as arrhythmia detection, at-home monitoring, chest band heart rate monitors, ECG monitors, respiration monitors, and wearable devices. In addition, it is optimized for dry electrodes, which is one of the key requirements for our specific

Table 1. Comparison of MAX3000x solutions (supply voltage 1.1–2 V, operating temperature 0–70 °C) [9–12].

Part Number	Biopotential		Bioimpedance	Supply Current (typical) [μA]
	ECG	Heart rate		
MAX30001	X	X	X	247
MAX30002			X	150
MAX30003		X		100
MAX30004	X	X		100

application. In this paper, we chose this front-end to measure ECG, as well as breathing from bioimpedance.

MAX30001 is available in a 30-bump wafer-level package (WLP). As shown in Fig. 4, it consists of a single biopotential channel providing electrocardiogram (ECG) waveforms and heart rate detection, and a single bioimpedance channel capable of measuring respiration [9]. For example, the ECG channel comprises an input MUX (which contains integrated several features such as electrostatic discharge (ESD) protection and electromagnetic interference (EMI) filter), a fast-recovering instrumentation amplifier, an antialiasing filter (AAF), and a programmable gain amplifier (PGA) [9].

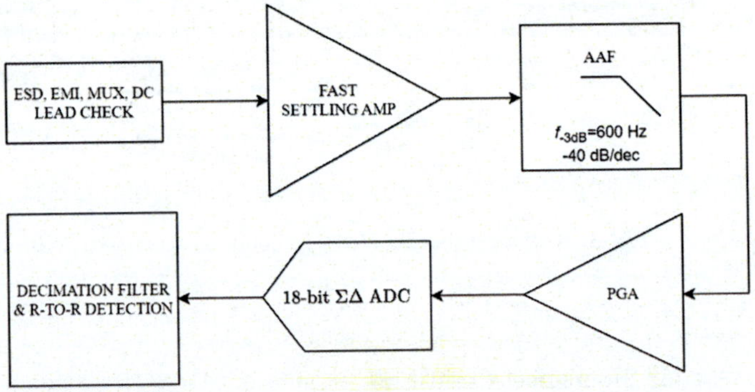

Fig. 4. MAX30001 ECG channel, simplified and adapted from [9].

Depending on the chosen operating mode, the first MAX30001 interrupt pin, assigned to the ECG channel, is configured to signalize either 16 samples threshold in the ECG FIFO buffer, its overflow, or the R-to-R detection of the ECG signal. ECG samples *ADC* are recorded in 18-bit resolution with 128 Hz sampling frequency and converted to voltage *VECG* via (1):

$$VECG[\text{mV}] = ADC * VREF/(2^{17} * ECG\_GAIN) \tag{1}$$

where *VREF* is the voltage reference (typically 1 V), and *ECG_GAIN* chosen 20 V/V gain [9].

The bioimpedance channel is similar to the ECG channel. Bioimpedance is sensed differentially and recorded in 20-bit samples *ADC* with maximum 64 Hz sampling frequency. Bioimpedance *BioZ* is then calculated by (2):

$$BioZ[\Omega] = ADC * VREF/(2^{19} * BIOZ\_CGMAG * BIOZ\_GAIN) \quad (2)$$

where *VREF* is voltage reference (typically 1 V), *BIOZ_CGMAG* chosen injected current of a maximum 96 μA and 128 kHz frequency, and *BIOZ_GAIN* chosen 20 V/V gain [9]. Furthermore, a special function is implemented to calculate the respiration rate every 30 s or 60 s. It applies a Butterworth band-pass filter, Blackman window, and RFFT (Real Fast Fourier Transform) to calculate current breaths per minute based on 1280 transmitted samples.

To transmit data, MAX30001 uses a serial peripheral interface (SPI). The maximum SPI serial clock (SCLK) frequency is 12 MHz. Data is strobed into the MAX30001 on SCLK rising edges in form of 4-byte packages – the first byte is a command word (7-bit address and a Read/Write mode indicator) followed by a 3-byte data word [9].

2.2 BLE Central Processing Unit

The chosen ultra-low power platform with 1.8 V power supply comprises an ARM 32-bit Cortex-M4 central processing unit (CPU) for application development, and a dedicated 32-bit ARM Cortex M0+ CPU for real-time radio layer and network protocols [13]. These two cores communicate via inter-processor communication (IPC) controller and hardware semaphore to prevent shared resource access conflicts (Fig. 5) [14].

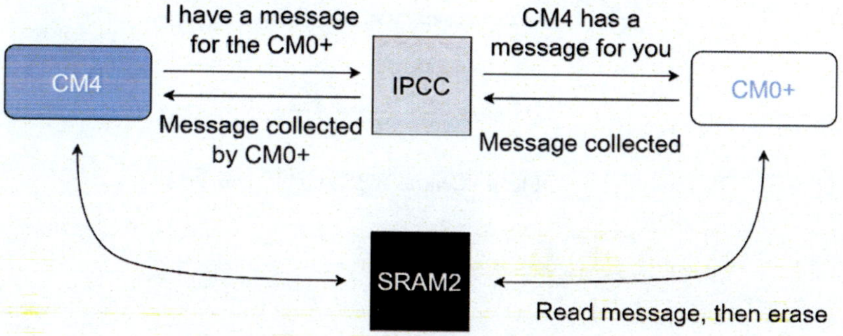

Fig. 5. Dual core operation, adapted from [13].

The used VFQFPN68 package version, with 1 MB flash memory, 256 KB SRAM and up to 64 MHz clock frequency, supports two protocols based on IEEE 802.15.4-2011 standard – Thread and Zigbee 3.0, as well as Bluetooth Low Energy 5.0 [13]. It will be used to establish communication with MAX30001 via SPI interface on one hand, and with a personal computer via BLE protocol on the other.

2.3 Wireless Body Sensor Node

The central WBS unit, designed as a four-layer PCB with dimensions of 25 × 41 mm, is shown in Fig. 6. The device is powered whether by a single Li-Po battery, whether by the USB power supply, which contains a pi filter and a battery charger. Moreover, the power supply circuitry contains overcurrent and overvoltage protection, accompanied by two switching regulators. Via SPI interface, MAX30001 transmits the measured data to the STM32WB55 microcontroller, which also establishes BLE communication as a FreeRTOS task. For the purpose of wireless communication, a 2.4 GHz mini SMT ceramic antenna with a 50 Ω matched network and a band-pass filter for harmonics removal is used. Apart from the aforementioned units, the WBS contains the ICM-20948 MEMS inertial motion unit (IMU) for motion tracking. Its use is for now for demonstrational purposes only. The desktop application was monitoring and data collection is designed in Python 3 language along with Qt tools, while the Android mobile application is implemented in C# language using the Xamarin platform.

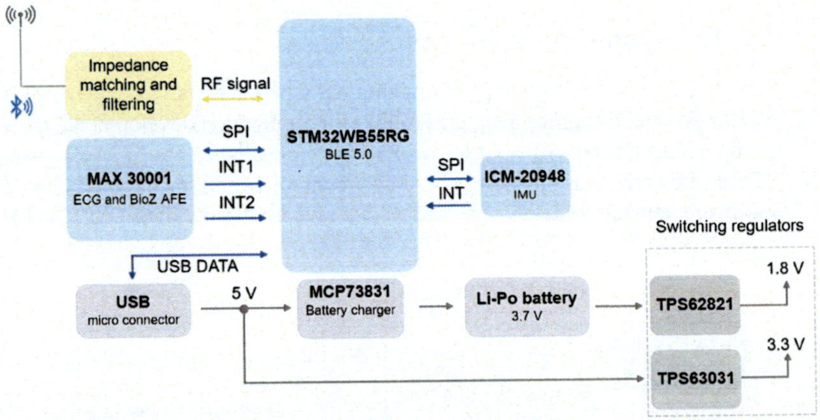

Fig. 6. Central WBS unit block diagram.

2.4 BLE Protocol

BLE Communication. When the implementation of BLE protocol is considered [6], the controller and host blocks are implemented on Arm Cortex-M0+, whereas the apps are implemented on Arm Cortex-M4 CPU. As mentioned before, the 2.4 GHz ISM band is used.

The entire BLE connection process is shown in Fig. 7. During advertising, the advertiser sends the packets at a fixed interval – from 20 ms up to 10.24 s in increments of 625 μs – via Primary Advertising Channels. The scanning device listens for advertisers, with or without sending scan requests in return. To establish a connection with the detected advertiser on the same physical channel, the scanning device, now called the initiator, sends a connection request packet. Above all, this packet contains information on frequency hopping sequence and connection interval. The latter parameter defines how often the devices will exchange data and ranges from 7.5 ms to 4 s, with a step size of 1.25 ms [7]. Now, the pairing can begin, during which the connected devices exchange keys to encrypt the link. Once they are paired, the initiator becomes the master, also known as GAP Central or GATT Client, whereas the advertiser becomes the slave i.e., GAP Peripheral or GATT Server [14].

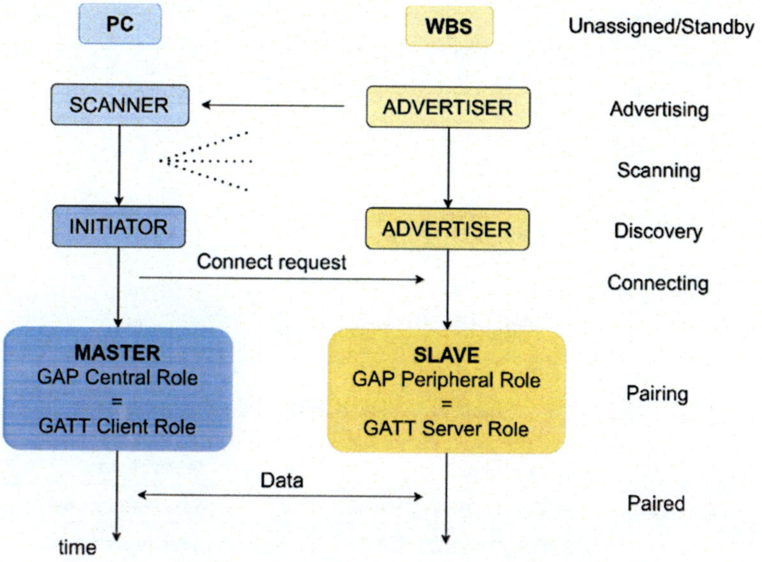

Fig. 7. Schematic of BLE connection process, adapted from [7].

BLE Implementation. BLE application is based on Cable Replacement public project from [15]. First, HAL (Hardware Abstraction Layer) STM32WB55 drivers are generated. With the use of STM32CubeMX tool, RTC, DMA, SPI, UART, USB, and RF interfaces, as well as input MAX30001 interrupt pins and output pins for LED indicators, are initialized. The USB interface is configured as a CDC (communications device class). Thus, acting as a USB-UART adapter, it allows STM32WB55 to be recognized as a virtual COM port able to establish serial communication with the personal computer. Afterward, ICM-20948 and MAX30001 are initialized via the SPI interface.

The initial graphical user interface (GUI), which is implemented in Python binding PyQt5, is shown in Fig. 8. Before initializing the BLE protocol, MAX30001 mode can be chosen via USB interface with STM32WB55, and option Configure. Altogether, 11 WBS modes are implemented, as listed in Table 2.

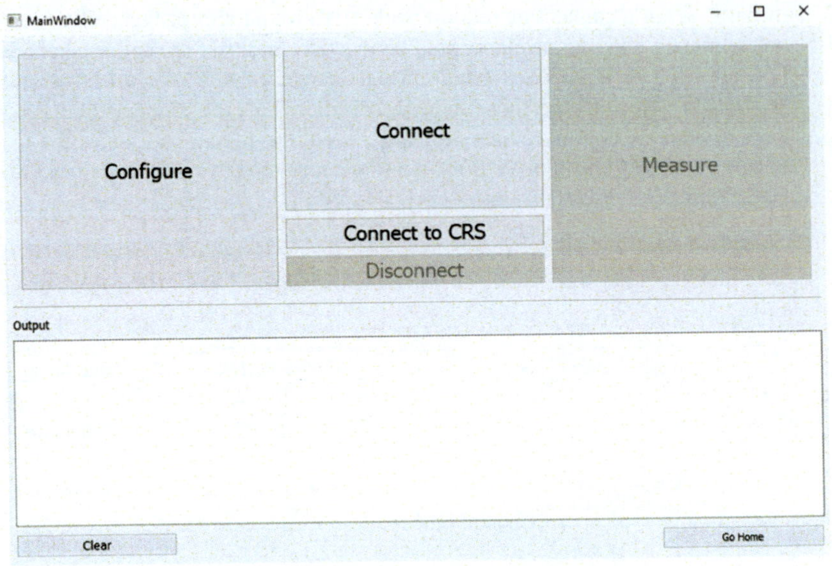

Fig. 8. Initial Python graphical user interface.

Table 2. Available WBS operating modes.

	Device mode	Description
MAX30001	ECG_OUTPUT_MODE	Send ECG signal
	RTOR_OUTPUT_MODE	Send heart rate
	HR_ECG_OUTPUT_MODE	Send EC signal and heart rate
	BIOZ_OUTPUT_MODE	Send bioimpedance
	BPM60_BIOZ_OUTPUT_MODE	Send bioimpedance, along with respiration rate every 60 s
	BPM30_BIOZ_OUTPUT_MODE	Send bioimpedance, along with respiration rate every 30 s
ICM-29048	ACCEL_OUTPUT_MODE	Send acceleration
	GYRO_OUTPUT_MODE	Send gyroscope data
	MAGN_OUTPUT_MODE	Send magnetometer data
	TEMP_OUTPUT_MODE	Send temperature
	COMBINED_OUTPUT_MODE	Send all ICM-29048 data combined

Next, Bluetooth Low Energy stack on Cortex-M0+ is initialized, along with the Host Controller Interface, GAP, and GATT. Then, the main Cable Replacement Service is created with its 128-bit Universal Unique Identifier (UUID). Lastly, the BLE advertising can begin.

By choosing the option *Connect* in GUI, scanning for nearby BLE advertisers begins. Once the device is detected, user must choose a BLE service to create connection. To automatically choose the correct device and service, the option *Connect to CRS* is available.

After the pairing process, the STM32WB55 task scheduler controls data acquisition and the BLE communication process, in accordance with the chosen device mode.

3 Results

In order to test MAX30001 and system performance, two test scenarios (TS) were devised and carried out.

TS1. The bioimpedance is measured with two common dry graphite electrodes placed directly on the chest in the fourth intercostal space (Fig. 9). Breaths per minute (BPM) were calculated for 3 min using BPM60_BIOZ_OUTPUT_MODE device mode. Each minute, the respiration frequency was increased. Results are shown in Fig. 10. According to recent researches, such as [16], respiratory rate can also be extracted from ECG signals. Since the bioimpedance measurement was carried out primarily for the purpose of respiration measurement, this means that future integration could focus solely on ECG signal acquisition. Of course, regarding the cycling application, bioimpedance measurement on the chest had entirely testing purposes.

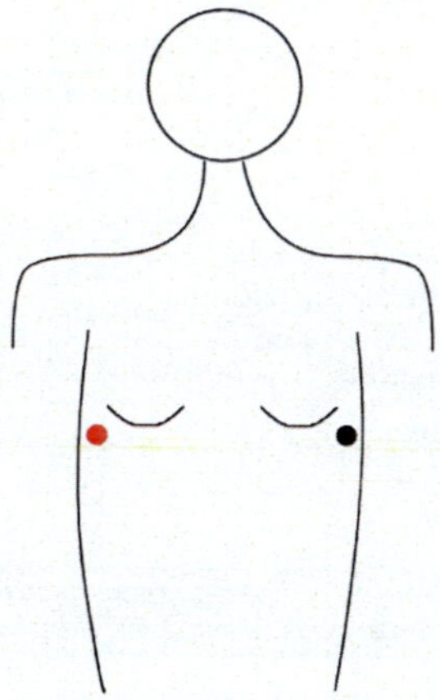

Fig. 9. Dry electrodes position for bipolar bioimpedance measurement.

TS2. To test the ECG signal reception as well, the system is thereafter implemented on a G6.1 bold FS electric bicycle from the *Greyp Bikes* company [17], as shown in Fig. 11.

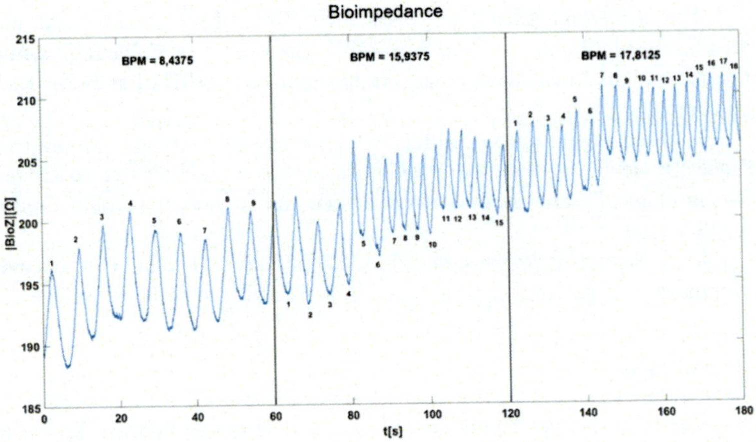

Fig. 10. Measured bioimpedance over the course of 3-min breathing with increasing frequency: 9 BPM, 15 BPM, 18 BPM respectively.

With two dry electrodes [8] with outer radius of 30 mm placed on handles, ECG signal was measured while the subject was pedaling in place. To obtain a sufficient signal-to-noise ratio (SNR), a third body bias dry electrode was placed on the dorsal side of the right hand. The results are shown in Fig. 12. Naturally, the ECG signal would be stronger if measured directly on the chest (closer to the heart), but such a configuration is not a practical solution for this kind of wearable application. To use ECG signals for both heart rate and respiratory measurements as mentioned earlier, an unbiased comparison of ECG signals for both scenarios would be crucial.

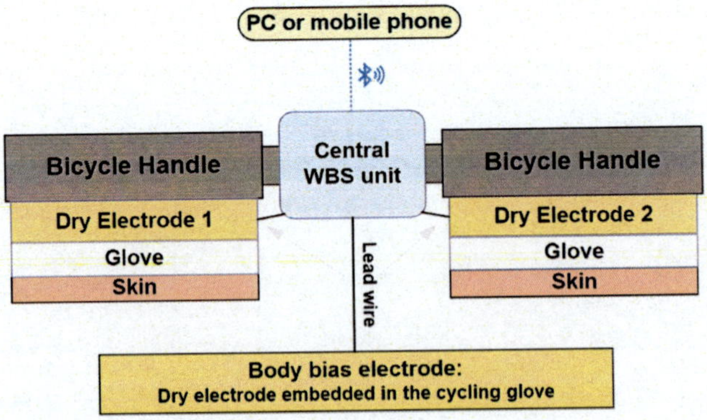

Fig. 11. ECG measurement system.

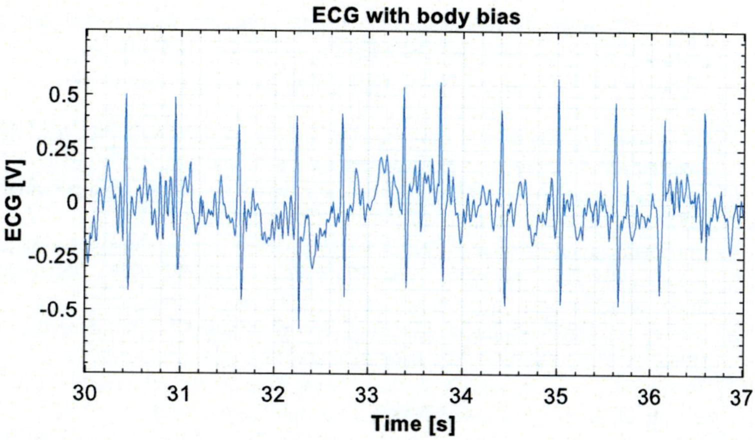

Fig. 12. Excerpt of an ECG signal recorded on thumbs with dry electrodes placed on bicycle handles.

4 Conclusion

Through bioimpedance and respiration, as well as ECG measurements, capabilities of MAX30001 are examined and confirmed. In combination with the Bluetooth Low Energy protocol, inertial motion unit, and STM32WB55RG platform, integrated wireless biomedical system is created. Furthermore, the developed system is successfully adapted for electric bicycles, thus proven to be suitable for wearable health monitoring applications. Future work will focus on further improvement of the coupling between the dry electrodes and cyclists' skin in order to achieve measurements without the third body bias electrode, and on signal processing possibilities in order to use ECG signals for both heart rate and respiratory rate measurements.

Acknowledgment. This research has been supported by the project "GMP – Greyp Micromobility Platform" (EFRR-IR-II grant KK.01.2.1.02.0027).

References

1. Perez, A.J., Zeadally, S.: Recent advances in wearable sensing technologies. Sensors **21**(20) (2021)
2. Wearables – statistics & facts. https://www.statista.com/topics/1556/wearable-technology/#topicHeader__wrapper. Accessed 29 Sept 2022
3. Naranjo-Hernández, D., Callejón-Leblic, M.A., Lučev Vasić, Ž., Seyedi, M., Gao, Y.-M.: Past results, present trends, and future challenges in intrabody communication. Wirel. Commun. Mob. Comput. (2018)
4. Negra, R., Jemili, I., Belghith, A.: Wireless body area networks: applications and technologies. In: The Second International Workshop on Recent Advances on Machine-to-Machine Communications 2016 (2016). Procedia Computer Science, vol. 83, pp. 1274–1281, Elsevier

5. Čuljak, I.: Wireless body sensor communication systems based on UWB and IBC technologies: state-of-the-art and open challenges. Sensors **20**(12) (2020)
6. What is Bluetooth Range? What You Need to Know. https://www.adorama.com/alc/bluetooth-range/. Accessed 22 Sept 2022
7. Catanzaro, D.: Study and investigation of bluetooth low energy security in the IoT environment, master thesis, Politecnico di Torino (2020)
8. Portelli, A., Nasuto S.J.: Design and development of non-contact bio-potential electrodes for pervasive health monitoring applications. Biosensors (2017)
9. Maxim Integrated Products: Ultra-Low-Power, Single-Channel Integrated Biopotential (ECG, R-to-R, and Pace Detection) and Bioimpedance (BioZ) AFE, MAX30001 datasheet, September 2019
10. Maxim Integrated Products: Ultra-Low-Power, Single-Channel Integrated Bioimpedance (BioZ) AFE, MAX30002 datasheet, March 2018
11. Maxim Integrated Products: Ultra-Low Power, Single-Channel Integrated Biopotential (ECG, R-to-R Detection) AFE, MAX30003 datasheet, November 2016
12. Maxim Integrated Products: Ultra-Low Power, Single-Channel Integrated Biopotential (R-to-R Detection) AFE, MAX30004 datasheet, December 2016
13. STMicroelectronics: Multiprotocol wireless 32-bit MCU Arm®-based Cortex®-M4 with FPU, Bluetooth® 5 and 802.15.4 radio solution, STM32WB55RG datasheet, November 2020
14. STM32WB Workshop v20. https://www.st.com/content/dam/AME/2019/stm32wb-workshops-2019/STM32WB_Workshop_Presentation.pdf. Accessed 22 September 2022
15. STM32CubeWB MCU Firmware Package. https://github.com/STMicroelectronics/STM32CubeWB. Accessed 29 September 2022
16. Liu, H., Allen, J., Zheng, D., Chen, F.: Recent development of respiratory rate measurement technologies. Physiol. Meas. (2019)
17. Greyp Bikes. https://www.greyp.com. Accessed 27 September 2022

Automatic Objective Magnification Detection in Brightfield Microscopy by Use of Neural Network

Dora Machaček[1](✉) and Ivan-Conrado Šoštarić-Zuckermann[2]

[1] Veterinary Faculty, University of Zagreb, Heinzelova 55, 10000 Zagreb, Croatia
dmachacek@vef.hr

[2] Department of Veterinary Pathology, Faculty of Veterinary Medicine, University of Zagreb, Heinzelova 55, 10000 Zagreb, Croatia

Abstract. In brightfield microscopy, commonly used digital cameras are still lacking many features that are required for high-quality digital images. Many of those features such as correction for geometric distortions, chromatic aberration, and vignetting are often done automatically by both professional and smartphone cameras. In scientific imaging, those in-camera corrections are even more essential but, in microscopy, they cannot be done automatically because information about the magnification and microscope objective is often not available to the camera. In this paper, we show that real-time artificial neural networks can be successfully used for the detection of objective magnifications in microscopy. We demonstrate that a real-time artificial neural network trained on only 8000 images can successfully classify four different objective magnifications of 4X, 10X, 20X, and 40X with 92% accuracy on previously unseen images. The approach that we put forward may enable manufacturers to implement these features into their microscopy cameras.

Keywords: Microscopy · Deep learning · Artificial intelligence

1 Introduction

In-camera lens corrections are widely used in the industry by all major camera manufacturers like Canon [1], Nikon [2], and Sony [3]. It is fundamentally impossible to make a perfect lens and these corrections are needed in order to offset certain lens imperfections that are, to a greater or lesser degree, present in every lens [4, 5]. The most common lens corrections are for optical vignetting [6], chromatic aberration [7], and geometric distortion [8]. Optical vignetting refers to a gradual loss of light intensity toward the image corners (see Fig. 1a). It naturally occurs in all optical systems and it is caused by intrinsic lens characteristics [9]. Chromatic aberration is a wavelength- dependent artifact that occurs due to lens inability to bring all of the wavelengths into a common focus. In microscopy, even the highest corrected, apochromatic objectives (corrected axially for all three main colors) can still suffer from lateral chromatic aberrations near the periphery of the field of view when white light illumination is used (see Fig. 1b).

P. Bonačić Bartolin et al. (Eds.): BioMedVetMech 2022, IFMBE Proceedings 90, pp. 73–80, 2024.
https://doi.org/10.1007/978-3-031-42243-0_7

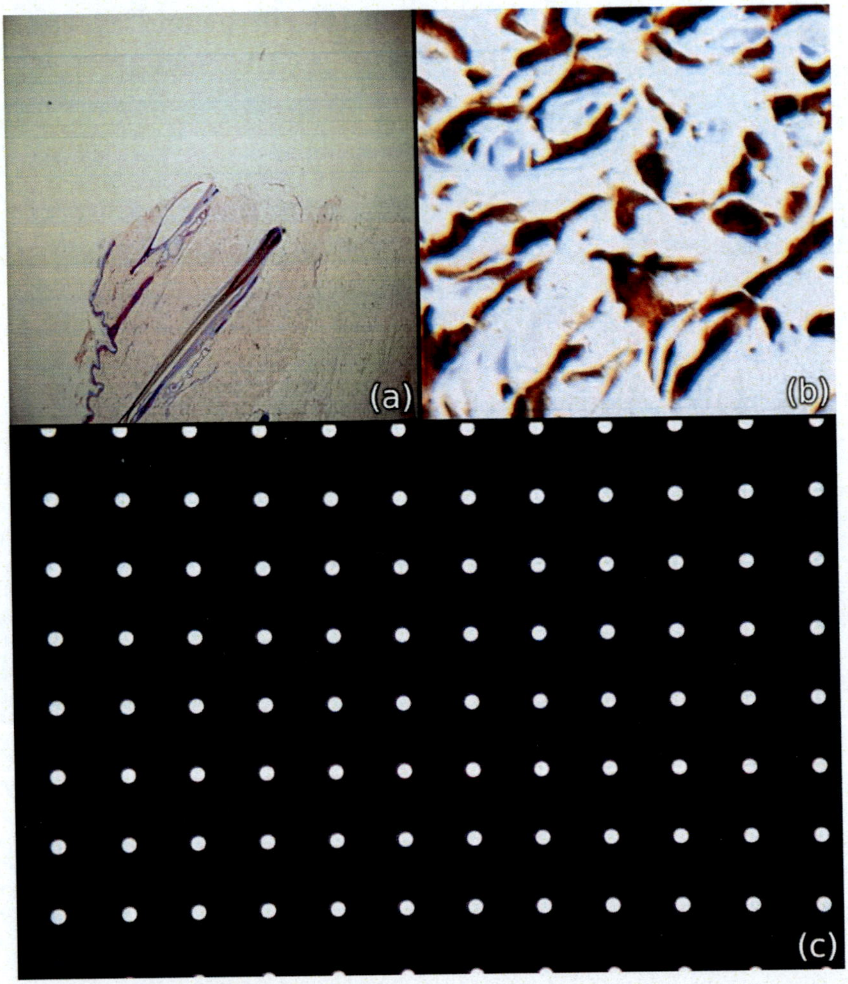

Fig. 1. Visualizations of optical vignetting (a), chromatic aberration (b), and barrel geometric distortion (c) aberrations.

Geometric distortion represents the change in shape (geometry) of the image (see Fig. 1c) and can represent a significant problem in microscopy, especially if various measurements from those images are later used in scientific publications. So, in our opinion, in order to get a scientifically accurate representation of objects under a microscope, these aberrations have to be corrected. Fortunately, they can easily be corrected without losing any significant information if an accurate lens correction model is known [10]. However, in conventional brightfield microscopy, that is rarely the case since information about the magnification and microscope objective is often not available to the camera, and thus, those corrections cannot be done automatically, without user input. To the best of our knowledge, there is no publicly available work on the automatic detection of microscope's objectives. In order to remedy that, we implemented a system that can automatically and accurately recognize which objective lens magnification is being used. In addition to aberration corrections, such a system can also be used to automatically put a scale bar on images for a publication.

2 Methodology

2.1 Data Collection and Creation

The dataset that was used to train our model was created using a BestScope BS-2082 brightfield microscope and a BigEye 10MP microscope camera. In total, we collected 10,000 images with four different apochromatic objectives: 4X, 10X, 20X, and 40X (2500 images per objective) from 80 tissue samples that were randomly selected from histopathology slide archive of Department of Veterinary Pathology, Veterinary Faculty, University of Zagreb. Images were splitted into four categories accordingly, and resized from their original size of 3704 × 2778 to 1024 × 1024 pixels using Python's OpenCV [11] INTER_LANCZOS4 interpolation functions. We divided the dataset into two sets and made sure that a single tissue sample does not end up in multiple sets. Eight thousand images were put in a training set and used to fine-tune a pre-trained model described below. In order to be able to measure the training success, 2000 images were set aside to form a so-called validation (DEV) set. The point of the validation set is to measure the model's performance on images that it has not "seen" during the training. However, since decisions on hyperparameter values are made based on the model's performance on the validation set, the final model's performance on the validation set will no longer be entirely representative of its real-world performance. Therefore, for the final evaluation of the model, one additional test set was created. However, in order to remove possible biases and make it more representative of real-world conditions, 4000 images for this set were collected by a different person, and with a different microscope with achromatic microscope objectives. Images were resized and splitted with the same criteria we used for a training set.

2.2 Model

We used PyTorch [12] official implementation of SqueezeNet v1.1 [13] neural network architecture with 720,000 parameters that was pre-trained on ImageNet-1k Dataset [14]. Pre-trained model was downloaded directly from PyTorch model Hub [15]. The motivation behind choosing SqueezeNet was its high throughput (Table 1) caused by its light architecture with few parameters.

All training experiments were done using a batch size of 32, Stochastic Gradient Descent [16] as an optimizer with a starting learning rate of 0.001 and momentum of 0.9. Learning rate was reduced by a factor of 0.1 every 7 epochs, for a total of 200 epochs. Models were trained on RGB images. We used Cross Entropy as a loss function. To select the best model, we simply took the best performing model on the validation (DEV) set, according to accuracy metric. All training and testing experiments were done on an Nvidia RTX 3090 GPU.

Tabel 1. FPS table: (on Nvidia RTX 3090 GPU and AMD Ryzen 9 5900X 12-Core CPU) In batched mode (sending batches to the model), pure inference (loading tensors into gpu + inference)

IMAGE SIZE	fps GPU	fps CPU
224 × 224	6000	300
512× 512	1100	40
1024× 1024	300	10

2.3 Augmentations

In order to increase the number of images we trained our model with, we used image augmentations. The images were slightly changed in a controlled manner without significantly changing the underlying content that would affect the ground truth labels. We employed the Albumentations [17] library for that purpose. Image augmentations have the following purpose: (1) to increase the diversity of data which leads to stable training, (2) increase the model's robustness to various effects that could be encountered in unseen data, and (3) decrease the chance of overfitting to spurious patterns in the data. As mentioned previously, every objective lens can display a different pattern of aberrations that are specific to that objective. For example, a model could easily overfit to the amount of vignetting, chromatic aberrations or even barrel and pincushion geometric distortion, therefore learning to differentiate between various aberrations instead of image magnifications. In addition to those aberrations, every objective lens has a different transmittance profile due to the different amount and type of glass used in the production of lens elements and the use of different lens coatings. This can change white balance and, more generally, image color profile – another lens characteristic a model can overfit on.

We trained models in three augmentation settings: plain (w/o), basic (B), and harsh (H). Plain setting refers to a training protocol without any augmentation, while basic and harsh settings differ only in the augmentations' occurrence probabilities, where under harsh setting, all augmentations have higher occurrence probabilities. We employed several types of augmentations: random brightness and contrast changes, channel shuffling, random hue and saturation changes, random gamma, per channel histogram equalization, and multiplicative noise in order to simulate changes in brightness, white balance, and exposure. Gaussian noise and ISO noise were used to simulate spurious dust and camera sensor effects, while optical distortion and vignetting simulated lens effects. Additionally, for standard image augmentations we opted for random flipping, random rotations by 90°, and small random rotations. Vignetting was implemented as a dot product of two gaussian kernels with shifting centers around the center of the images. The resulting kernel was scaled and multiplied with the image.

3 Results

We tested our model with three different image sizes: 224 × 224, 512 × 512 and 1024 × 1024, under three different settings: no augmentations (plain), basic augmentations and harsh augmentations. Since splits are class-wise balanced, we choose accuracy as a main evaluation metric. We also provide sensitivity and specificity for each class label.

Table 2. Model inference results on 224 × 224 sized images. DEV = validation dataset; ACC = accuracy.

SETTING	DEV	TEST			
	ACC	ACC	MAGNIFICATION	SENSITIVITY	SPECIFICITY
w/o	0.9860	0.5010	4x	0.3541	1.0000
			10x	0.0000	0.0000
			20x	0.7342	0.1160
			40x	0.9403	0.8891
B	0.9780	**0.8255**	4x	0.8244	0.9176
			10x	0.7622	0.7095
			20x	0.7593	0.8580
			40x	1.0000	0.8138
H	0.9590	0.7856	4x	0.8093	0.8372
			10x	0.7197	0.6798
			20x	0.6986	0.8900
			40x	0.9972	0.7322

In Table 2 we can see that models trained with augmentations are performing much better on 224 × 224 sized images. The best-performing model is trained with basic augmentations, while the worst-performing is the plain model. The Plain model failed to correctly classify any of 10X images and has poor performance on 4X images (only 35.41% sensitivity) and on 20X images (only 11.60% specificity). To identify why the plain model failed on the first three classes, we can check sensitivity and specificity, where it is clear that the model actually learned to classify only the last class (40X) and simply overfitted on the rest, what is confirmed with a high accuracy on the validation (DEV) set and a low accuracy on the test set. We believe that it happened because valuable information was lost during the process of resizing, so the model diverged from the global optimum. Fortunately, that problem is partially solved by simple augmentation, which is confirmed by decent performance of our augmented models on the test set.

In Table 3, we can observe that as information loss decreased, the plain model's accuracy almost doubled (80%), whereas the other models increased in performance only slightly, around 10%. A similar trend follows in Table 4 where the plain model's performance increased by 15% and other models stagnated because the model either did

Table 3. Model inference results on 512 × 512 sized images. DEV = validation dataset; ACC = accuracy.

SETTING	DEV	TEST			
	ACC	ACC	MAGNIFICATION	SENSITIVITY	SPECIFICITY
w/o	0.9900	0.7946	4x	0.6214	1.0000
			10x	0.7930	0.4012
			20x	0.9199	0.8500
			40x	0.9911	0.9289
B	0.9890	**0.9018**	4x	0.8815	0.9693
			10x	0.8807	0.8458
			20x	0.8672	0.9140
			40x	0.9976	0.8745
H	0.9810	0.8794	4x	0.8448	0.9904
			10x	0.8394	0.8676
			20x	0.8693	0.8380
			40x	1.0000	0.8138

Table 4. Model inference results on 1024 × 1024 sized images. DEV = validation dataset; ACC = accuracy.

SETTING	DEV	TEST			
	ACC	ACC	MAGNIFICATION	SENSITIVITY	SPECIFICITY
w/o	0.9910	**0.9267**	4x	0.8908	1.0000
			10x	0.9403	0.8715
			20x	0.8973	0.9440
			40x	0.9976	0.8870
B	0.9870	0.9088	4x	0.8756	0.9981
			10x	0.9343	0.9269
			20x	0.8600	0.9340
			40x	1.0000	0.7657
H	0.9880	0.8993	4x	0.8727	0.9981
			10x	0.9114	0.9150
			20x	0.8505	0.9100
			40x	0.9973	0.7636

not have enough capacity or it reached its local optimum. Overall, the best-performing model is the plain model trained on 1024 × 1024 images (Table 4), which further highlights that it is important to preserve as much information as we can in magnification classification tasks.

4 Discussion and Conclusion

Even though, to the best of our knowledge, there are not any studies about the classification of objective magnification in brightfield microscopy, we implemented a system that can automatically and successfully classify four different objective magnifications. The main takeaways of our study are: (1) there is important information in greater resolution images so we should not always down-sample the images in order to decrease inference time, and (2) augmentation helps (up until a certain point). We showed that as we increased the image resolution, the model that has not been trained on augmented images gradually improved, whereas the augmented models stagnated at 512 × 512 resolution. We believe that the inflection point happens at 1024 × 1024 resolution where the most important information is preserved even for a 4X objective and the model converges towards a different but better local optimum. To test that hypothesis and gather more insights, we plan to extend our testing data with completely different tissue types not seen in our training and validation sets. Further increase in the performance should be achieved by gathering more images, which is a common practice in Computer Vision.

Our paper demonstrates that a real-time artificial neural network can successfully classify different objective magnifications with high accuracy and thus enable manufacturers easier implementation of aberration corrections into their camera system.

References

1. Canon. https://www.canon-europe.com/pro/infobank/in-camera-lens-corrections/. Accessed 3 Oct 2022
2. Nikon. https://downloadcenter.nikonimglib.com/en/download/fw/348.html. Accessed 3 Oct 2022
3. Sony. https://www.sony.com/electronics/support/articles/00016553. Accessed 3 Oct 2022
4. Ahmed, M., Farag, A.: Nonmetric calibration of camera lens distortion: differential methods and robust estimation. IEEE Trans. Image Process. **14**(8), 1215–1230 (2005)
5. Hughes, C., Glavin, M., Jones, E., Denny, P.: Review of geometric distortion compensation in fish-eye cameras. In: IET Irish Signals and Systems Conference, ISSC (2008)
6. Kordecki, A., Palus, H., Bal, A.: Practical vignetting correction method for digital camera with measurement of surface luminance distribution. SIViP **10**, 1417–1424 (2016)
7. Kaufmann, V., Ladstädter R.: Elimination of color fringes in digital photographs caused by lateral chromatic aberration. In: XXth International CIPA Symposium, Italy (2005)
8. Wonpil, Y.: An embedded camera lens distortion correction method for mobile computing applications. IEEE Trans. Consum. Electron. **49**(4), 894–901 (2003)
9. Emery, W., Camps, A.: Introduction to Satellite Remote Sensing: Atmosphere, Ocean and Land Applications. 1st edn. Elsevier (2017)
10. Weng, J., Cohen, P., Herniou, M.: Camera calibration with distortion models and accuracy evaluation. IEEE Trans. Pattern Anal. Mach. Intell. **14**(10), 965–980 (1992)

11. Bradski, G.: The OpenCV library. Dr. Dobb's J. Softw. Tools (2000)
12. Paszke, A., Gross, S., Massa, F., Lerer, A., Bradbury, J., Chanan, G., et al.: PyTorch: an imperative style, high-performance deep learning library. In: Advances in Neural Information Processing Systems 32, pp. 8024–8035. Curran Associates, Inc. (2019)
13. Iandola, F.N., Han, S., Moskewicz, M.W., Ashraf, K., Dally, W.J., Keutzer, K.: SqueezeNet: AlexNet-level accuracy with 50x fewer parameters and $<$0.5MB model size. arXiv:1602.07360 (2016)
14. Deng, J., Dong, W., Socher, R., Li, L.-J., Li, K., Fei-Fei, L.: ImageNEt: a large-scale hierarchical image database. In: 2009 IEEE Conference on Computer Vision and Pattern Recognition, pp. 248–255 (2009)
15. Pytorch Hub. https://pytorch.org/hub/. Accessed 3 Oct 2022
16. Ruder, S.: An overview of gradient descent optimization algorithms. arXiv:160904747 (2016)
17. Buslaev, A., Parinov, A., Khvedchenya, E., Iglovikov, V.I., Kalinin, A.A.: Albumentations: fast and flexible image augmentations. arXiv:1809.06839 (2018)

Virtual Surgery and 3D Printing in Craniofacial Surgery – Our Experience at UHC Osijek Using a Newly Developed Add-On for "Open-Source" 3D Modeling Software

Vjekoslav Kopačin[1,2](✉), Ivan Mumlek[3], Vedran Zubčić[3,4], Josip Butković[1,2,3,4], and Luka Šimić[1,2,3,4]

[1] Department of Diagnostic and Interventional Radiology, University Hospital Center Osijek, Josipa Huttlera 4, 31000 Osijek, Croatia
vkopacin@gmail.com

[2] Faculty of Medicine, Department of Biophysics and Radiology, Josip Juraj Strossmayer University of Osijek, Josipa Huttlera 4, 31000 Osijek, Croatia

[3] Department of Maxillofacial and Oral Surgery, University Hospital Center Osijek, Josipa Huttlera 4, 31000 Osijek, Croatia

[4] Faculty of Medicine, Department of Otorhinolaryngology and Maxillofacial Surgery, Josip Juraj Strossmayer University of Osijek, Josipa Huttlera 4, 31000 Osijek, Croatia

Abstract. With the advancement of medical technologies, especially imaging technologies, and the further advancement of computer systems, advanced visualization techniques, including 3D printing and virtual or mixed reality is the logical next step in medical imaging of pathology. Their implementation enables clinicians more personalized approach to patient treatment. Therefore, the production of personalized surgical guides is becoming a standard. Since the "in-house" development of the Add-On FFF Gen for open-source CAD software Blender at the end of 2019, from 2020 until now, 11 patients underwent the successful surgery of the mandible reconstruction with "free fibula flap" using 3D printed personalized surgical guides. An increase in the number of cases treated in such a way, and good postoperative results only confirm the advantages of the application of these methods in everyday clinical work.

Keywords: Computer-aided Design · Medical informatics applications · Printing (three-dimensional) · Virtual surgery · Mandibular reconstruction · Free fibular flap

1 Introduction

Due to the large number of important structures located in a small place, head and neck surgery, especially reconstructive surgery, can be extremely complicated, time-consuming, and exhausting for surgeons [1]. In the conventional approach to mandibular reconstruction, every osteotomy, including position and angle, is based on the surgeons'

P. Bonačić Bartolin et al. (Eds.): BioMedVetMech 2022, IFMBE Proceedings 90, pp. 81–87, 2024.
https://doi.org/10.1007/978-3-031-42243-0_8

experience and the final decision is made intraoperatively [2]. The results could be imprecise and affected not only the appearance but also the patient's functioning in everyday life.

With the advancement of medical technologies, especially imaging technologies, and the further advancement of computer systems that are available in everyday clinical practice, advanced visualization techniques, including 3D printing and virtual or mixed reality are logical next step in medical imaging of pathology, and their implementation enables clinicians more personalized approach to patient treatment. By introducing 3D printing in more complex operations, surgeons have the opportunity for better preoperative planning and to go to the operating room with a clear idea of the extent of mandibular resection, the size and shape of the fibular bone fragments, and the fitting of the osteotomy. Restoring facial contour after tumor resection is one of the main goals after ablative surgery and fitting osteotomies is integral in the process.

A number of articles describe how virtual surgical planning and the use of three-dimensional (3D) printed models and surgical cutting guides could be useful in reducing operative time and visual outcomes [3–8].

The production of surgical cutting guides still lies largely in the domain of commercial biomechanical engineering companies whose services must be outsourced and can be expensive. There are commercial software available, but they come at a higher price. Dell'Aversana Orabona et al. [7] showed that low-cost, 3D-printed, "in-hospital" surgical guides have as good postoperative results as using commercially available computer-aided design (CAD) software or cutting guides, opening up the possibility of a personalized approach to the treatment of complicated cases in hospitals in less wealthy, transition countries that do not have large budgets. This is the reason why we developed an Add-On for open-source 3D modeling software, Blender.

2 Blender Add-On: FFF Gen

As mentioned in the previous section, the production of surgical cutting guides still lies in the domain of commercial biomechanical engineering companies or using commercial software whose price is also costly, delaying implementation of the 3D printing technologies in everyday use. There are reported successful cases in the production of personalized surgical guides using open-source 3D modeling software Blender like Ganry et al. [8] and Numajiri et al. [9], but the end users need to be proficient in the use of 3D CAD software Blender in order to produce good results consistently.

Unlike workflow described by Ganry et al., and Numajiri et al., where measurements of the distances, angles, and all 3D modeling are mostly done manually, our approach provides a framework where surgical guides can be produced using a set of relatively simple 3D operations (a combination of translating, rotating and scaling objects in 3D space). The more advanced operations, such as parenting and setting up Boolean operations, osteotomy plane angulation, etc. are hidden behind newly implemented operators and this is in more detail described in our previously published article [10].

Compared to other mentioned methods, FFF Gen Add-On provides a faster workflow, as cutting-guide modeling time is reduced compared to other authors who report times of 50 min or higher [7, 8]. The most important factor, the method is simplified so the end-users (surgeon, radiologist, or radiology technician) don't have to be proficient in 3D CAD software as many hospitals still do not employ biomechanical engineers. Additionally, as changes in graft dimensions are observed in real-time, this framework also serves as a tool for "virtual surgery" and visualization of the resulting guides and fibula grafts.

3 Our Experience in UHC Osijek Using In-House Developed Blender Add-On FFF Gen

The Add-On was developed at the end of 2019. The first case of mandibular reconstruction surgery, where personalized surgical guides designed with FFF Gen Add-On were used, was performed in January 2020. Since then, personalized cutting guides were designed for a total of 15 patients (Table 1) by two persons: cutting guides for the first case were generated by an Add-On developer and the rest by the radiologist at UHC Osijek. Of those 15 cases, 11 (73.33%) patients underwent surgery where personalized guides were used, two were operated on without surgical guides, in one patient had surgery canceled due to improper native site blood vessels status and possible bad outcome of the flap, and one patient decided to be treated in another institution. 7 patients were male and 4 were female. The average age of surgically treated patients using the personalized guides is 50.7 $\pm$ 11.6 years (youngest 36 y. o., oldest 71 y. o.).

The cause of the mandibular defect in 8 patients was a malignant tumor (gingival carcinoma), three had benign tumors (two mandibular ameloblastoma and one odontogenic keratocyst).

In 8 cases right fibula bone with a skin flap was chosen as the donor site mostly due to surgeons' preference in workspace organization and surgical approach. During preoperative planning in the rest of the patients, using CTA images and CAD 3D models of fibulas and lower limb arteries, it was decided to harvest the left fibula bone and skin flap because of the unfavorable anatomy or atherosclerotic disease of the peroneal artery.

In 9 patients, two bone segments (4 osteotomies) of the fibula were used in mandibular angle and body reconstruction, and in two patients one bone segment was used (two osteotomies).

Outsourced service was used for 3D printing of the surgical guides, using biocompatible polymers (Stratasys Objet 30 3D printer and VeroGlaze MED 620 resin). Overall turnaround time of the initial CT scanning to the cutting guides sterilization was less than one week.

Using affordable FDM 3D printer Prusa i3 MK3, anatomical models of the patient's native mandible were 3D printed and used in preoperative planning and prebending of osteosynthesis plates. For 5 (33.3%) cases, more than one model was 3D printed: in two cases model of the mandible was printed together with a matching tumor, in one case native mandible was 3D printed together with a previously placed osteosynthesis plate, and in one case, a because of large bone defect, the native mandible was 3D printed with mirrored mandible model used for prebending of the osteosynthesis plate, and in one case together with the model of the mandible, surgical guides were printed for "mock-up" surgery.

Assessment of the bone fragment alignment during the surgery and bone fragment healing on follow-up images used a qualitative visualization method that relied on the expertise of the most experienced surgeon in the team with about 20 years of experience in this type of mandibular reconstruction surgery.

Table 1. Summary of the mandibular reconstruction surgeries with free fibula flap performed with the FFF Gen Blender Add-On since January 2020 at UHC Osijek, Croatia.

	Total No. of Cases	No. of Surgically Treated	Patients Males Females
Mean patient age (SD)	52.9 (11.5)	51.6 (11.1)	49.3 (14.0)
Cause of the reconstructive surgery			
Malignant tumor	10	4	3
Benign tumor	4	2	1
Other	1	0	0
Virtual surgery and FFF Gen application	15	7	4
Donor site fibula			
Right	11	4	4
Left	4	3	0
Median No. of bone fragments	2	2	2
Median No. of osteotomies	4	4	4

4 Discussion and Conclusion

The osteocutaneous free flap, when treating defects of the mandible, became standard for complex oromandibular reconstruction following resection of tumors, as well as osteomyelitic and osteonecrotic parts of the mandible [11]. Restoring facial contour after tumor resection is one of the main goals after ablative surgery. As said earlier, conventional surgeries of mandibular resection and its reconstruction are based on surgeons' experience and the final decision is made intraoperatively [2]. The results can be imprecise, requiring the surgeon to perform additional corrections like bone fragment edge abrading, bone fragments angle corrections etc. which further prolongs the duration of the operation and tires the surgical team. Also, unsatisfactory mandibular arch reconstruction could impair not only the appearance but also the patient's functioning in everyday life.

With the introduction of advanced visualization techniques and 3D printing into UHC Osijek's Department of maxillofacial and oral surgery for more complex surgeries like the one above discussed, surgeons have the opportunity for better preoperative planning and go into the operating room with a clear idea of the extent of tumor resection, size, and shape of fibular bony fragments and fitting osteotomies as seen in Fig. 1.

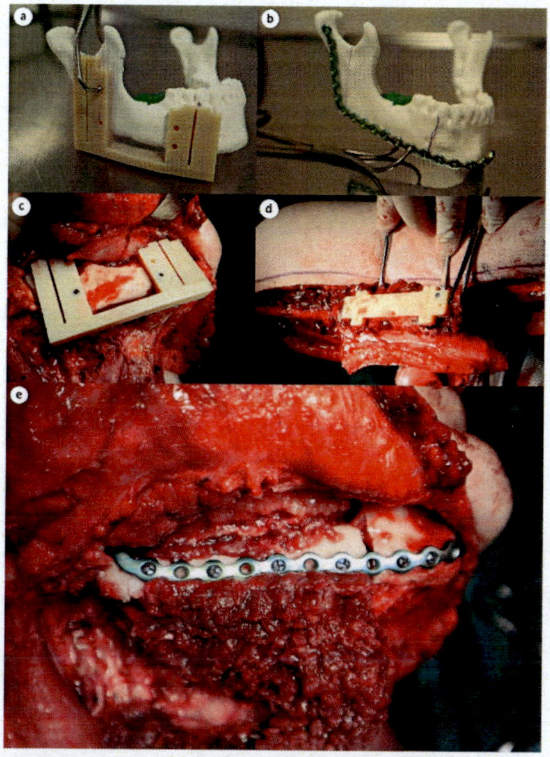

Fig. 1. a. trying the fitment of the surgical cutting guide to the 3D printed preoperative model of the patient's mandible and tumor. b. prebending of the osteosynthesis plate on the 3D printed model of the patient's mandible. c. and d. the perfect fit of the guides to the mandible and fibula; cutting planes match the width of the osteotomy saw (the width can be adjusted as needed in one of the steps in Add-On) and the surgeons only need to follow the predetermined plane for matching fibular bone fragment as seen on e. e. excellent fitting of the flap's bone fragment to the native mandible.

In the example of our three patients, using conventional and advanced visualization methods, this also came to the fore when, during the preoperative planning, we changed the operative plan, i.e. the harvesting place of the free flap due to anatomical variation of the arteries or heavy atherosclerotic burden that could impair free flap function.

In our experience, preoperative 3D planning and the use of cutting guides can make a surgeon's life a lot easier. With precise osteotomies at the desired site, made with personalized cutting guides, the final result is better, while in the cases before the usage of the surgical guides, osteotomies were not so precise leading to the appearance of the bone spurs that needed to be manipulated additionally, i.e. burred. The bone fragments heal faster and better meaning there is less space between the graft and the healthy mandible as seen in Fig. 2. According to the most experienced maxillofacial surgeon in the team, satisfactory reconstruction of the mandible was achieved in 6 patients meaning there is a complete union of the bone fragments in the follow-up scans (orthopantomogram and CT scan), in one patient there is a 2,5 mm gap between two bone fragments, which is still satisfactory result and for three patients there are no feedback as patient are being followed in an-other medical institution. In one patient due to the progression of the primary tumor in interval time between virtual surgery and cutting guides design and actual surgery, a mismatch between previously designed guides occurred, but surgeons used previously agreed cutting angles, and widened the bone fragment, thus achieving satisfactory mandibular arch reconstruction.

One of the key elements is the extent of resection and with the use of preoperative planning and virtual surgery, the surgeon doesn't have the burden of altering the treatment plan during the surgery. On the other hand with the use of cutting guides, both in resection and on the donor sites, the end result is far more predictable than before, when cutting guides were not used. With all modalities combined, in the end, the patients get far better results, which they deserve, and are more satisfied with their final appearance as seen in the Fig. 2c.

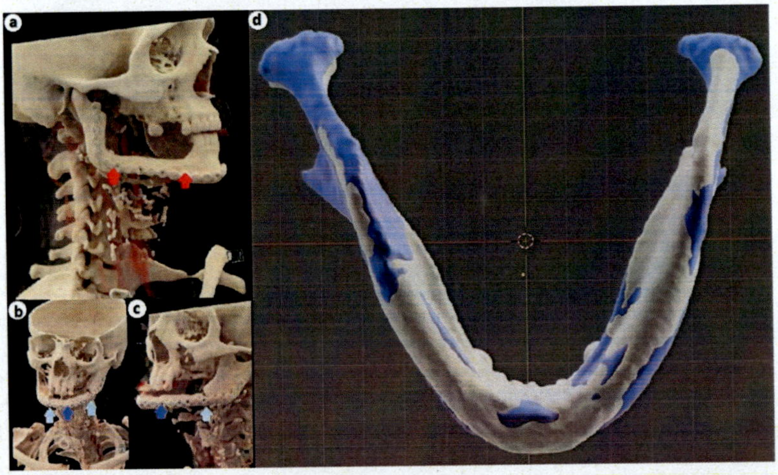

Fig. 2. Cinematic Rendering reconstructions in two patient CT scans. a. a routine follow–up CT scan performed 13 mo. After the surgery in a 38 y. o. the female patient (the same patient from the Fig. 1.) shows the complete union of the single bone graft (red arrows) with the rest of the native mandible. b., c. and d. follow–up CT scan 22 mo. After the mandibular reconstructive surgery in a 68 y. o. the female patient shows restored mandibular arch with excellent aesthetic properties seen in b., and a closer view in c. shows the complete union between two bone grafts (dark blue arrows) and very good union between both bone fragments and native mandible (light blue arrows). d. overlay display of the two 3D models in the same patient: a preoperative 3D model seen in white color and a postoperative 3D model seen in blue color, showing a perfectly restored mandibular arch after the reconstructive surgery performed with personalized surgical guides designed with FFF Gen.

The good results achieved by applying advanced visualization methods and 3D printing in the fibula free flap mandibular reconstructive surgeries at UHC Osijek further strengthened the foundations and encouraged surgeons to continue using this technique mandibular defects reconstructions and even other regions of the head and neck. In the future, there is a possibility of a step forward in terms of installing dental implants in the same act, also using appropriate personalized guides as well as developing similar open-source Add-Ons for other reconstructive bone microvascular surgery in the head and neck region.

References

1. Pellini, R., Mercante, G., Spriano, G.: Step-by-step mandibular reconstruction with free fibula flap modelling. Acta Otorhinolaryngol. Ital. **32**(6), 405 (2012)
2. van Zyl, O., Fagan, J.: Atlas of otolaryngology, head & neck operative surgery free tissue transfer flaps in head & neck reconstruction: microvascular anastomosis technique (2015)
3. Prisman, E., Haerle, S.K., Irish, J.C., Daly, M., Miles, B., Chan, H.: Value of preoperative mandibular plating in reconstruction of the mandible. Head Neck **36**(6), 828–833 (2014)
4. Azuma, M., et al.: Mandibular reconstruction using plates prebent to fit rapid prototyping 3-dimensional printing models ameliorates contour deformity. Head Face Med. **10**(1), 1–8 (2014)
5. Poukens, J., Haex, J., Riediger, D.: The use of rapid prototyping in the preoperative planning of distraction osteogenesis of the cranio-maxillofacial skeleton. Comput. Aided Surg. **8**(3), 146–154 (2003)
6. Jacek, B., et al.: 3D printed models in mandibular reconstruction with bony free flaps. J. Mater. Sci. Mater. Med. **29**(3), 1–6 (2018). https://doi.org/10.1007/s10856-018-6029-5
7. Orabona, G.D., et al.: Low-cost, self-made CAD/CAM-guiding system for mandibular reconstruction. Surg. Oncol. **27**(2), 200–207 (2018)
8. Ganry, L., Hersant, B., Quilichini, J., Leyder, P., Meningaud, J.P.: Use of the 3D surgical modelling technique with open-source software for mandibular fibula free flap reconstruction and its surgical guides. J. Stomatol. Oral Maxillofac. Surg. **118**(3), 197–202 (2017)
9. Numajiri, T., Nakamura, H., Sowa, Y., Nishino, K.: Low-cost design and manufacturing of surgical guides for mandibular reconstruction using a fibula. Plast Reconstr. Surg. Glob. Open **4**(7) (2016)
10. Šimić, L., Kopačin, V., Mumlek, I., Butković, J., Zubčić, V.: Improved technique of personalised surgical guides generation for mandibular free flap reconstruction using an open-source tool. Eur. Radiol. Exp. **5**(1), 1–6 (2021). https://doi.org/10.1186/s41747-021-00229-x
11. Lin, P.-Y., Lin, K.C., Jeng, S.-F.: Oromandibular reconstruction: the history, operative options and strategies, and our experience. Int. Sch. Res. Not. **2011** (2011)

Author Index

B
Bašić, Silvio 19
Brnić, Dragan 1
Butković, Josip 81

C
Cifrek, Mario 53, 60
Čuljak, I. 60

D
Demarin, Vida 19
Đerke, Filip 19
Džapo, H. 60

K
Klaić, L. 60
Kopačin, Vjekoslav 81
Kostešić, Petar 1
Krešić, Nina 1
Krizmanić, Severino 35

L
Lasić, Slaven 19
Ljolje, Ivana 1

M
Machaček, Dora 73
Mumlek, Ivan 81

N
Naletilić, Šimun 1

P
Papeš, Dino 35
Pavić, Predrag 35
Peharec, Stanislav 53
Popović-Maneski, Lana 46
Prišlin, Marina 1

S
Šajinović, P. 60
Šimić, Luka 81
Šoštarić-Zuckermann, Ivan-Conrado 73
Srhoj-Egekher, Vedran 53
Stanešić, A. 60

T
Turk, Nenad 1

V
Virag, Zdravko 35
Vlahović, Dunja 1
Vrhoci, I. 60

Z
Zubčić, Vedran 81

P. Bonačić Bartolin et al. (Eds.): BioMedVetMech 2022, IFMBE Proceedings 90, p. 89, 2024.
https://doi.org/10.1007/978-3-031-42243-0